from
MADNESS
to
mindfulness

Advance Praise for
From Madness to Mindulness

"Gunsaullus's mindfulness practices and analysis will appeal to any woman interested in practical approaches for maintaining emotional and sexual health, as well as to readers confronting and dealing with shame."

— *Publishers Weekly*

"Dr. Jenn Gunsaullus has created an amazingly down-to-earth roadmap of sexual mindfulness that takes you from discovery to practice. I don't know a woman who wouldn't identify with Jenn's story or benefit from her process. Even though mindfulness is a constant in my advice to Ílisteners, it's still something I need to remind myself about all the time, and I know this book will not only help me, but help others begin their journey on a more sexually mindful path."

— Dr. Emily Morse,
founder and host of the *Sex with Emily* Podcast
and SiriusXM Radio Show

"Educational and empowering. Gunsaulles' new book challenges readers to think differently about women and sex, and provides a roadmap to their authentic sexual selves."

— Dr. Justin Lehmiller,
research fellow at The Kinsey Institute and author of
Tell Me What You Want

"I was hooked from the first word to the last. This book speaks directly to countless women I have counseled for issues related to sex and intimacy. It is an insightful page-turner that is loaded with practicality and compassion. This book is a game-changer! I truly believe that *From Madness to Mindfulness* will help many women to make peace with their relationship with their sexual selves."

—Neil Cannon, Ph.D., LMFT.
sex therapist, couples counselor, professor of
Marriage & Family Therapy, Denver Family Institute

"Gunsaullus writes with a rare freshness that brings alive her message that women can heal the split between shame and pleasure through a mindfulness approach. She offers everyday solutions to the crisis of unworthiness and sexual discomfort among females today, and shows women how to embrace their pain, feel their vulnerabilities, and soothe their aching souls to become fully empowered sexual humans. This book is a must-read for those who are flailing to find ballast in these confusing times about sex, dating and relationships. Dr. Jenn provides a practical road map for women to navigate ways for thriving in this new sexual world."

— Patti Britton, PhD, AASECT
past-president, clinical sexologist,
co-founder of SexCoachU.com

"With deep compassion, Dr. Gunsaulles challenges societal messages that commonly stand in the way of women's sexual fulfillment and provides practical solutions. *From Madness to Mindfulness* is a loving how-to for anyone seeking greater self-awareness, pleasure, and self-sexual discovery."

—August McLaughlin,
author of *Girl Boner* and host of Girl Boner Radio

"I am very impressed with Dr. Jen's ability to put into such clear words what so many people experience. Her book is thought provoking and a perfect read for anyone just beginning their personal journey of sexual self empowerment. I will be recommending this book to clients and look forward to more work by her."

—Dr. Laurie Bennett-Cook,
clinical sexologist and director of Sex Positive Los Angeles

"This book reminds readers that, yes, self-care, personal growth, and good sex matter — and that everyone deserves good sex! Dr. Jenn's Reinventing Sex Plan is sure to help anyone looking to reinvent more than just their sexual world."

—Dr. Tammy Nelson,
certified sex therapist and author of
Getting the Sex You Want and *The New Monogamy*

"Honest, fun, and far-reaching, this book challenges us, as women, to think of ourselves and our intimate relationships in a new way – with practical guidance at each step of the process. Dr. Jenn does a masterful job of defining the components of mindfulness; weaving meaningful scenarios from her own life story, with pertinent client vignettes – and applying her own philosophy and recommendations to all aspects of the female sexual narrative. I find each chapter a vital tool for reflection – to enhance one's own awareness, express our truths, and ultimately transform our experience of relationship."

—Debra Wickman, MD, FACOG, NCMP, CSC,
gynecologist, sexuality counselor, and Founder/CEO
of Fantastically Female, LLC

"Dr. Jenn Gunsaullus gives us so many gems and brilliant one-liners — on nearly every page I found myself slapping my hand on the table while reading, saying "YES! THIS!" or pausing to take notes. *From Madness to Mindfulness* is both a well-articulated philosophy on sexual wellness and an actionable step-by-step guide for women who want to transition to a state of sexual happiness, fulfillment, and authenticity in their lives. Dr. Jenn is a master at disarming difficult topics like toxic masculinity, rape culture, religion, vulnerability, body image, and sexuality, and at utilizing compassion to help you along your sexual journey. I cannot wait to recommend *From Madness to Mindfulness* to my clients!"

—Dr. Jill McDevitt,
sexuality educator and sexual wellness coach

"Being able to tune into yourself and your partner is a key element of great relationships and amazing sex. *From Madness to Mindfulness* gives you plenty of tools and skills to make it happen, along with down-to-earth tips and ideas for creating the best relationships possible. With lots of the simple and practical ideas and an honest perspective on sex and gender, this book is a must read."

—Charlie Glickman PhD,
sex & relationship coach

"Jennifer Gunsaullus, PhD has written a book guiding the way out of those familiar self-defeating messages about our bodies and our sexuality that, no matter her age, every woman has heard for much of her life. Using mindfulness, meditation, and other carefully illustrated exercises, she shows us the way for a woman to dump internalized negative beliefs, reclaim her power, and enjoy her sexuality without shame."

—Isadora Alman, MFT, CST,
columnist at Psychology Today, author of
What People Keep Asking Me About Sex & Relationships

from
MADNESS
to
mindfulness

Reinventing Sex for Women

Jennifer Gunsaullus, PhD

CLEiS
PRESS

Published in the United States by Cleis Press, an imprint of Start Midnight, LLC, 101 Hudson Street, Thirty-Seventh Floor, Suite 3705, Jersey City, NJ 07302.

Printed in the United States.
Cover design: Allyson Fields
Cover photograph: Pexels
Text design: Frank Wiedemann
First Edition.

10 9 8 7 6 5 4 3 2 1

Trade paper ISBN: 978-1-62778-296-8
E-book ISBN: 978-1-62778-509-9

TABLE OF CONTENTS

· · · · ·

To my parents,
for your unconditional love, support,
and humor.

INTRODUCTION

I was sitting in the dark near the back of one of the fourth-grade classrooms. Some of our moms were there, including mine, along with our teachers. Well, the *female* fourth-grade teachers. The boys were in another classroom, with the one male teacher. I don't know what they were doing; nobody talked about it. We, however, were watching a cartoon about menstruation, and at the age of ten, this was the first time I was hearing about it.

The movie was biology-based, with nothing overtly graphic. Nonetheless, it was not sitting well with me. What the hell was this thing that was going to happen to me? I started feeling warm and uncomfortable in my chair; I tried to distract myself by listening to the *flip, flip, flip* of the projector. I'd never felt this kind of visceral, slow-building nausea, although I was no stranger to carsickness.

I was wearing my favorite red sweater, a button-down that I wore as a cape with only the top button fastened. But even so, it was too warm. I took it off. I started taking deep breaths. I stared at the tiled pattern on the floor, willing myself to be okay. *You're fine. You feel okay. Really, you're fine.*

Then I threw up. All over the floor. And I started crying. The lights came on, but I saw nothing. The next thing I remember is sitting outside on the wooden bench on the elementary school's front porch, doubled over crying. My mom was calmly telling me that I probably wouldn't have to worry about getting my period for another few years.

Even in writing this story, some thirty-four years later, I feel the hollowness of humiliation in my heart and solar plexus, and a rising warmth and light-headedness from shame. But over the years, I've gained skills in how to sit with this kind of discomfort and not allow it to shut me down.

● ● ● ● ●

This book is for the many women who have internalized the madness of negative messages in small ways or big ones. By "madness," I mean the huge and continuous barrage of conflicting and undermining messages we girls and women receive about our sexuality and bodies. *You're too fat, too skinny, too tall, too short, too muscular, too weak, too pale, too dark, too slutty, too prudish* . . . and the list goes on. There is always something wrong with us, which we may hear from parents, partners, the media, strangers on the street, or our own inner dialogue. We are taught to dislike ourselves, viewing *me* as the enemy.

Sex is complicated. Although its innate purpose is procreation, we all know it has a lot of other meanings and purposes, such as pleasure, fun, and connection. "Sexuality" refers to the full experience of being a sexual person, including beliefs, experiences, attractions, emotions, neurochemicals, activities, and pleasure. Unfortunately, so many women in the United States struggle to enjoy their own sexuality. In addressing this problem, we often ask the wrong questions and, therefore, arrive at the wrong solutions. Then the problem is perpetuated and unwittingly passed down to each generation. With the continual messages we receive, urging us to dislike our bodies and feel shame about our sexual expression or lack thereof, it is the rare woman who experiences an active, healthy, expressive, and satisfying sex life in a long-term relationship. But there is hope; this book is about reinventing sex for women.

I believe that rather than focusing on pleasure or the inability to achieve pleasure, we must first focus on discomfort. This does not sound sexy, but please, follow along with me. In order to experience a depth of pleasure and satisfaction, women must first explore and understand the negative messages around sex and their bodies that they learned growing up, and lean in to this discomfort. In fourth grade when I threw up at the thought of a period, I didn't have the skills to sit with the discomfort and then process it through in a healthy way. I was left with shame and embarrassment about my body, menstruation, and the whole experience. Most of us have a lifetime of such uncomfortable experiences around our sexuality, experiences that build up over time and create a barrier to satisfying sexual interactions.

When I use the term "sit with the discomfort," I'm referring to the ability to notice uncomfortable thoughts or emotions, articulate what they are (to yourself or another), accept that the discomfort is happening in that moment even if you don't like it, and choose to notice all of that instead of shutting it out or distracting yourself. This process might sound confusing, terrible, or impossible! But I assure you, it's quite possible, quite empowering, and a skill I will be teaching throughout this book.

There's a lot of advice out there about how to reinvent your sex life. But the media's focus on "How to have more powerful orgasms" or "Pleasing your partner in ten new ways" is simplistic and unrealistic for better sex because it only looks at half of the equation—pleasure. It ignores the importance of understanding the thoughts, emotions, and feelings about sex that may be scary and uncomfortable—the real source of women's concerns. Throughout this book, I'll discuss this idea of noticing your thoughts and emotions and choosing to focus your attention on them—what I call "staying present." In our pill-popping, magic-bullet society, we are often sold simple solutions that distract us from our discomfort. However, the solution to sexual issues is to do the difficult work of creating a deeper understanding of ourselves. This means being aware at new levels we may not have known were possible. Exploring nuances of self-awareness has the potential to help those of us who feel sexually disempowered, confused, or unhappy. With such mindfulness, we can all create our own version of sexuality that is personally empowering.

If you are a woman who is totally comfortable with your sexuality and body, if you move with ease and mindful awareness in sexual situations and communication, if you are comfortable being vulnerable both emotionally and physically, and if you love yourself deeply, then this is not the book for you. And as a side note—congratulations! You have managed to create inner strength, comfort, and expression as a sexual woman, despite potent media messages to the contrary. That is something to be celebrated!

However, I believe most of us in the United States are learning, experiencing, and expressing female sexuality in ways that don't work for us. We may simply want to know what a normal sex life is and how to fit into that norm. But what if the norm is a messed-up, unhappy, and unfulfilled sex life? Because that *is* the norm for many women. *Normal* doesn't sound so appealing now, does it?

But we can change that.

THE IMPORTANCE OF SELF-WORTH

Five women of various ages sat in a circle in uncomfortable folding chairs. At thirty-one, I appeared to be the youngest there. The small room was just a few steps off the sidewalk, and I glanced up as a group of teenagers walked, chatting, past our open door, perhaps just enjoying the sunny Sunday afternoon, or more likely, walking to the nearby Starbucks for a caffeine and sugar fix. "Please close your eyes now," our workshop facilitator instructed, pulling my attention back to the group. I didn't really like her so far—she had what felt like a faux-spiritual personality—but I had paid my twenty bucks, so I was going to get the most out of my two hours. We Gunsaulluses are a frugal people.

The leader, her voice calm and monotone, continued. "Place your hand over your heart. Concentrate on opening your heart center. Think about what you love about yourself. Imagine it . . . Visualize it . . . Feel it . . ." I started thinking about how proud I was that I had driven cross-country alone, that I appreciated how quickly I was able to make new friends, that I loved spending time with my boyfriend, that . . . that . . . *Uh oh. Damn it! Why are there tears again? I don't want to cry in front of these strangers!*

As I continued to visualize what I liked about myself, and felt a lightness of gratitude and joy in my chest, those feelings quickly mixed with a dampening pressure on my heart. I had no control over my flowing tears.

A few minutes later we were asked to open our eyes.

"Who would like to share?" our facilitator asked gently.

I knew that I should share about my experience with the group. I had been quiet so far, and it was clear something was going on for me now. I could feel the burden of expectation from the group. Or at least I thought I could. I had been reading about and practicing mindfulness for a few months, since moving to San Diego, and I was taking this women's workshop for personal growth and empowerment. But the dancing, prickly feeling in my solar plexus and the nausea in my belly—bodily sensations I would learn in later years meant I had a fear of feeling embarrassed and being judged—had kept my lips sealed. Yet without another thought I now raised my hand.

"You can probably see my tears." The words tumbled out of my mouth, as I looked around the room, avoiding eye contact. "I'm not sure why this happens, but in the past couple of months, every time I meditate on self-love, I start crying. So clearly something is going on. I think I feel sad thinking about self-love because there are parts of me I don't love."

Acknowledging this made me cry harder, as the other participants looked at me through kind eyes.

This would be the first of many public vulnerability moments for me, as my personal growth led me along a new path into mindfulness and authenticity.

● ● ● ● ●

I was raised a "good girl" in a small town in Pennsylvania, outside of Philadelphia. I was outspoken at a young age, with a sense of fairness and kindness, especially around perceived injustices (e.g., a classmate picking on the new boy in class). But I also followed the rules of being a good girl, in terms of being obedient and not rocking the boat. At a young age I had internalized messages about the danger of getting pregnant from sex. I was a responsible kid.

In November of 1991, my freshman year at Lehigh University, I recall watching the television in my dorm room when Magic Johnson announced that he was retiring from basketball because he was HIV positive. This announcement propelled conversations about HIV and AIDS to a new level in the United States. The good girl in me heard the hidden message loud and clear: Sex was not just irresponsible, it could be deadly. By the end of my sophomore year, I had joined the campus club for sexual health peer educators; we presented condom demonstrations and sexually transmitted disease prevention workshops on campus. I was quickly intrigued by gender differences in sex and sexual decision-making and the power dynamics that seemed to exist between women and men in the sexual realm.

I went on to graduate school at the State University of New York at Albany, and my research for my PhD dissertation in sociology focused on HIV prevention programs and adult women's sexual health education. I traveled to five cities around New York State to interview educators in community-based organizations (CBOs) who worked to halt the spread of HIV in their local communities. This was the early 2000s, when the spread and impact of HIV and AIDS in ethnic-minority communities was finally being recognized by government agencies with funding for education. I was thirty years old, educated, white, suburban-raised, nonreligious—a woman visiting CBOs primarily located in poorer black, Latino, or Asian immigrant city neighborhoods. The educators were mostly members of the communities they served, and some were HIV positive. They kindly opened their doors to me, engaging in interviews about their educational efforts and allowing me to observe their community HIV prevention workshops. These visits to CBOs and community spaces were an invaluable aspect of my professional and personal growth.

Thirty-six educators answered my questions about a variety of topics related to culture, gender, power, religion, and safer sex. Among other questions, I asked, "If you only had time to stress one thing regarding sexual health or prevention for women, what would that be?" The responses really surprised me. From my sexual health education training in college and graduate school, I assumed the primary answer would pertain to condom use. A few educators did say something along those lines, but the majority said they would emphasize self-worth, self-esteem, self-love, and the need for women to nurture or prioritize themselves. I didn't understand this at first. How was that going to help with preventing HIV? But this was the seed for me to recognize that at the core of overall sexual health is our feeling of worthiness.

Think about it this way: If you don't think you're good enough or worthy enough to avoid HIV, why would you ask your sexual partner to use a condom or to discuss sexual health? Why would you care enough to take care of yourself, or even believe you have the ability to do so? Why would you ask for your needs to be met?

After completing my field interviews and defending my dissertation proposal, I moved to San Diego, California, to complete my analysis and writing from afar in much warmer and sunnier weather. The timing was fortuitous in terms of understanding these confusing responses about self-love and self-worth. In San Diego, I joined local holistic health groups and mind-body-spirit communities, and attended classes in mindfulness, meditation, yoga Reiki, energy work, life coaching, and personal transformation. Exposure to these new ways of thinking and moving through the world, based on mindfulness, compassion, authenticity, and vulnerability, was both terrifying and liberating. I came face to face with my own fears around self-love and self-worth. And I finally started to understand what those educators already knew: Self-worth is necessary for a healthy and fulfilling relationship and sex life.

Author and researcher Brené Brown, PhD, headquartered at the University of Houston, writes and speaks widely about issues of vulnerability and self-worth. In her research she discovered, quite unexpectedly, that shame is a heavy emotion that undermines worthiness—and lack of worthiness feeds shame. She writes, "Shame is basically the fear of being unlovable—it's the total opposite of owning your story and feeling worthy. In fact, the definition of shame that I developed from my research is: Shame is the intensely painful feeling or experience of believing that we are flawed and therefore unworthy of love and belonging."[1] Ironically, because Brown personally struggled with and resisted her own

---

1   Brené Brown, *The Gifts of Imperfection: Let Go of Who You Think You're Supposed to Be and Embrace Who You Are* (Center City, Minn.: Hazelden, 2010), 39.

vulnerability, she was dismayed by her own research, which found that allowing oneself to feel vulnerable was the key to real happiness. Having the courage, compassion, and connection to practice vulnerability is the only way to build worthiness.

In all my work with women who are dealing with sexual issues, from individual and couples coaching to small group workshops and large lectures, worthiness is at the crux of my work. So many of us are undermined and sucked into belief systems that put us in constant battle with our bodies and our sexuality. But if we claim our worthiness—take it as a fact—instead of basing it on performing to appease others, we suddenly have time and space to just be ourselves.

How do we claim our worthiness when we have so many external messages and internal beliefs that discourage it? The best way I have learned to move through shame to worthiness, and to practice the courage, compassion, and connection that Brown speaks of, is through full-body mindfulness.

MY PERSONAL INTRODUCTION TO MINDFULNESS

The first time I learned about mindfulness was in January 2004, having moved to San Diego from the Northeast two months earlier. San Diego has a thriving holistic health and yoga community, so in the spirit of "when in Rome," it wasn't long before I attended my first meditation class. Plus, I had made a promise to myself that I had to keep.

Our instructor guided the class of six or so to find comfortable seats on cushions, then to close our eyes for her guided mindfulness meditation. I felt like a fish out of water. I kept peeking to see what others were doing

and how they looked. One young man stood out to me—
he looked like a "good meditator" because of his erect
posture and apparent focus. To my surprise, no one else
was peeking. I guessed I was supposed to trust the situation and just go along with it. In retrospect, I realize I
was feeling silly and afraid to embarrass myself by doing
something "wrong" in a new environment. Now I look
forward to opportunities to practice calm awareness in
the community of others.

Why did I seek a mindfulness meditation class in the
first place? The three months leading up to my cross-
country move had been stressful. In the chaos of moving
from my apartment in Albany back to my parent's house
in Pennsylvania, meeting a new boyfriend, completing
my dissertation fieldwork, defending my proposal, and
delaying my San Diego move by a month to get everything
done, I experienced strong chest pains. I knew the cause
was anxiety, but the pain really hurt. I also knew that
deep breathing and visualizations could help, but I had
little practice in cultivating these skills. I made a promise
to myself that I would never again allow emotional stress
to cause physical pain in such a way. One of my goals in
moving to California—the la-la land of fruits and nuts,
right?—was to explore some "New Age" ideas and learn
how to reduce my anxiety and feelings of being overwhelmed. I was definitely in the right place.

Over the years I've learned that mindful awareness is
the foundation for all of my personal growth, and in the
long run, it has helped me feel happier and calmer. I've
learned to exercise choice in moments when I did not know
I even had options—and I consider that the epitome of
empowerment. In the short run, though, from battlefield

to battlefield, such awareness can feel scary, confusing, painful, and deeply uncomfortable. It is this discomfort, and learning how to stay present with this discomfort in new ways, that has been my path to living a life of intention and choice. This path has been so very different from the reactivity and programming that previously ran the show, with behaviors that proved problematic in my relationships, intimate interactions, and life overall.

WHY THIS TOPIC

As I was completing my dissertation, I started teaching small spiritual sexuality workshops for women in my home, and I continued my personal training around mindfulness by attending a five-day retreat with the world-renowned mindfulness teacher Thich Nhat Hanh. The next year I delved into the personal transformation classes of Landmark Education and conducted interviews with thirty-five women about their sexuality as part of one of my class projects. (I've pulled two relevant questions from these interviews and shared their responses in chapter 6.) At this point, some friends and acquaintances started asking if I would coach or counsel them around their sex, dating, and gender concerns. In this way, I was making a transition from graduate studies in academia to my own version of applied sociology in the sex and gender realm, and using mindfulness as the core of this approach.

In December of 2012, I channeled all these topics of interest into my first TEDx talk, *Sex: Mind Full or Mindful?*[2] This talk explored the state of female sexuality

2   You can watch *Sex: Mind Full or Mindful?* here: youtu.be/ neH09fTkNB4

in America and offered mindfulness tools for women to reclaim their sexual experiences and power. The positive feedback from men and women, both at the event and afterwards, further confirmed that I had struck a chord in our culture's zeitgeist. People saw how women were trained to dislike and disconnect from their own bodies and sexual experiences, and how mindfulness offered a new path for healing and growth. A couple years later I gave a second TEDx talk[3], this one about how various examples of female sexual disempowerment around the world are all linked to shame, and how this emotion controls women's minds and bodies. My workshops, coaching practice, TEDx talks, and all of the subsequent feedback led me to write this book to explore the themes of female sexuality, desire, shame, mindfulness, and community responsibility.

WHY SEX MATTERS

Sex is powerful. People sometimes do really foolish things in the sexual realm, primarily because it validates that they are attractive, desirable, worthy, or powerful. Think about powerful politicians or religious leaders who lost their careers because of their sexual secrets, which were often in direct opposition to how they told others to live. Their sexuality—their need to be sexual, experience eroticism, express their sexual desires, or perhaps prove their masculinity (or femininity) through sexual conquest—drove them to risk it all. Because sexual energy is so powerful, it can bring out the worst *and* best in us.

---

3   You can watch *Female Sexual Shame Hurts Us All* here: youtu. be/40riTBK9Qjo

When it is respectful, chosen, and connected, it gives us a feeling of joy. Audre Lorde, the late author and poet, spoke about the importance of erotic energy for women: "It is an internal sense of satisfaction to which, once we have experienced it, we know we can aspire. For having experienced the fullness of this depth of feeling and recognizing its power, in honor and self-respect we can require no less of ourselves."[4]

Good sex matters. It can matter in obvious ways, like creating and maintaining a healthy relationship, or it can matter in more nuanced ways, like as a way to be more vulnerable, and therefore intimate, with a partner. In this book, I speak to the self-knowledge and self-worth that have been taken away from many women regarding sexuality, or were never allowed to blossom in a conscious way in the first place. The topic of sex can elicit such discomfort, shame, and fear that it remains in the shadows of everyday life. Big emotions and fears around sexuality can fester and take on a life of their own. These get in the way of healthy, intimate relationships. This book shines a bright light on these topics so each of us can create a version of sexuality that works for *us*.

Whether you have thought much about the role of sex in your life or not, at some point in your life you will likely be with a partner who considers sex to be an important way to connect with you and to experience intimacy. Considering your partner's needs and how to negotiate with them while also being true to yourself is an important balance to achieve. For you women who are in

4   Audre Lorde, *Sister Outsider: Essays and Speeches* (Berkeley, Calif.: The Crossing Press Feminist Series, 1994), 54.

long-term relationships that involve only obligatory once-a-week or holiday sexual encounters, I know that your pleasure is not a priority or seems like an impossibility. But even if you view sex as an obligation, you deserve to have sexual experiences that are at least pleasant, and *even* pleasurable. For you, and for those across the full spectrum of sexual enjoyment and expression, this book will help expand your choices and experiences and help you create a version of sexuality that empowers you to live a happier and healthier life.

HOW TO USE THIS BOOK

This book will lead you on a journey of self-discovery by helping you cultivate your insight, inspiration, self-knowledge, and self-awareness. When relevant, I share specific stories from my clients and workshop participants. My clients have ranged from eighteen to eighty-two years old, and have included women and men; cisgender and transgender folks; those who identify as straight, bisexual, queer, and lesbian (since female sexuality is one of my main specialties, I tend not to attract gay men!); and people who are black, Latino, Asian American, Middle Eastern, and white. I've also had clients from a variety of religious beliefs, including Mormon, Protestant, Catholic, Baha'i, Jewish, Buddhist, self-defined spiritual, and atheist. I've given workshops or lectures in a variety of settings, including universities, women's health conferences, CEO events, yoga studios, senior centers, Mensa conferences, and various nonprofits. All of these interactions have shaped this book.

A note on language: when I use the term "woman," "girl," or "female," I'm referring to a person who identifies as female. When I use the term "man," "boy," or "male," I'm referring to a person who identifies as male. Sexuality experts agree that sex and gender are a spectrum, and that our traditional binary language of "male" and "female" does not accurately reflect the reality of experience for many individuals, including those who might identify as gender nonbinary, intersex, or transgender. However, for the purposes of this book, the cultural constructs and societal messages I'm discussing are based upon these traditional beliefs about binary sex and gender roles, as well as traditional stereotypes of femininity and womanhood. There is a specific set of messages in our culture targeting those who are raised female and/or identify as female, and for the most part, those are the ideas I am examining in this book. It's my sincere hope that as our understanding of sexuality and gender becomes more nuanced as a nation, the very gendered stereotypes I address in this book will become obsolete.

Chapter 1 explores sociological research into the "madness" surrounding female sexuality—the messages, contradictions, and confusion. You may have thought that the issues described here were specific to you, part of your personal struggle. But in this chapter, I will explain how such messages, contradictions, and confusion create a much larger set of sexual problems for women.

Chapter 2 introduces the concept of mindfulness, a powerful tool in addressing these problems. I show how and why mindfulness training is beneficial to your health and well-being and why it is so damn hard to be mindful sometimes. I also offer simple practices to integrate into your everyday life.

Chapters 3 through 5 apply mindfulness to specific areas of your personal life: healthy relationships and communication, sexual desire and passion, and body image. These are heavy topics for many women, and they fluctuate in importance through different phases of your lifetime. Cultivating mindfulness builds resilience to handle struggles from the past and new struggles as they emerge. The calmer, more appreciative, and more worthy you feel, the better prepared you are to weather your changing body, relationships, needs, and roles over time. These chapters are replete with suggestions to help you integrate mindfulness into your routines and relationships, and to improve your communication effectiveness, your ability to feel sexual desire, and your appreciation of your body.

Chapter 6 centers on compassion and service and the responsibility I believe we have to help younger generations of women feel empowered. This includes teaching ourselves and younger women how to clearly see the impact of the media on our self-worth. To break the cycle of female sexual disempowerment, we must offer our girls a new narrative rather than recreate patterns from our past. This new clarity can lead to a sisterhood based on collaboration, compassion, and responsibility.

At the conclusion of each of these chapters is a Reflection & Writing worksheet to help you move from passively reading to actively reflecting and doing. This type of reflection is so important for self-knowledge, greater awareness, and personal growth. I hope you'll find the questions stimulating and fascinating. I strongly suggest that you take the time to write out your answers, either in the space provided or in a journal. There is also an Action Item to guide you from reading and reflection on to action. You can tap the real power of applied mindfulness by paying attention to your thoughts, emotions, and bodily sensations while completing each chapter's worksheet.

While these chapters are packed with ideas and suggestions, you may still find it difficult to turn ideas into action. Chapter 7 outlines common roadblocks to growth, along with ways for you to get and stay motivated. Forming new habits requires structure and small, step-by-step daily efforts. I'll walk you through creating your own *Reinventing Sex* plan with practical daily, weekly, and monthly commitments to put the lessons learned in previous chapters into action. From daily reminders and appreciations to accountability partners and monthly checklists, I'll help you create a personalized plan for healing, expression, and connection. I also include the most current information on my website and social media (go to www.DrJennsDen.com to find all of this) to assist you in your personalized plan, and to create a tribe environment to support you as you heal, grow, and move forward on your mindful journey toward sexual happiness and health.

Chapter 8 will give you a boost as you begin your journey—a journey that requires courage. It takes guts to acknowledge personal flaws and commit to living differently. You must be brave to authentically own your fears as a sexual woman, and then move through those fears to happiness. While the effort may feel daunting, it *is* possible for you to plot a new sexual journey. By reflecting on societal sex messages that do not serve you and choosing to shift from those beliefs to feelings of worthiness, self-love, and self-acceptance, you can become a thriving sexual being *on your own terms*. When you reinvent your sexuality from a mindful perspective, the new and beautiful possibilities are limitless.

CHAPTER 1

SEX MADNESS

It was her second coaching session with me. She had come to see me because a few of her girlfriends had seen me already, and she was struggling with how to create healthy dating relationships. She had a warm smile and long, dark brown hair, and wore a tight, low-cut T-shirt.

I particularly enjoy working with her demographic: young, single women in their twenties who are committed to spirituality and personal growth. They are like sponges soaking up new and empowering ideas, and it is rewarding to see them grow and change.

As this young woman sat on my beige microfiber sofa, I asked about her homework assignment, about the reasons why she has sex. She started to cry. I paused a moment to give her space with her emotions as I sipped green tea from my Wonder Woman mug. Then I gently asked, "What's going on?"

"I realized that almost all the times I've had sex in the past two years, it was because it was easier to go along with it than to say no." She looked down at the floor, and she explained that she would meet guys at bars, enjoy talking and flirting with them, and end up going back to their place. She liked the attention. She liked feeling sexy and beautiful. They would start fooling around, and although she would be attracted to the guys, be aroused, and enjoy the sexual interactions, she did not want to have sexual intercourse right away. But the guys seemed to expect it, so she went along with it. She didn't get a lot of enjoyment out of the sex and didn't feel comfortable making requests about her needs. She felt like she was doing it for them—guys she had just met. But she blamed herself.

I moved the box of tissues closer to her in case she wanted one, and then I took one for myself. I felt my heart expand in empathy with her struggle and vulnerability. I knew she was not alone. This kind of sexual situation happened a lot more than most people knew, and sex and sexuality are complicated topics.

MADNESS FOR WOMEN IN AMERICA

You are not alone. If you are uncomfortable, judgmental, disillusioned, or even disgusted with some part of yourself or your sexuality, you are not alone. You're actually in quite good company with the majority of girls and women in the United States. It's important for you to realize that this does not mean there is something actually *wrong* with *you*. Your difficult experiences with parts of your body, your sexuality, or intimate feelings are part of the larger fabric of all social leanings in our society. It's not just you. And you're not crazy.

After a workshop I conducted with a *The Vagina Monologues* performance group a few weeks prior to their shows, a San Diego State University student wrote to me, "I liked that the workshop brought a lot of issues about self-judgment and shame to my attention. I felt relief that most of my/our insecurities come from really messed-up ideals rather than something that was actually wrong with me or us as women." She had previously assumed there was something wrong with *her* because of the discomfort she had with discussing sexual topics and her belief that her body wasn't good enough. It's vital to our personal growth to know that we've been taught a lot of harmful things about our sexuality, but those messages don't mean we are bad, wrong, or broken. One of the reasons we don't know this is because we are also taught to stay quiet.

Speaking up and speaking out is generally uncomfortable for women. Brené Brown, researcher extraordinaire on the uncomfortable topics of shame and vulnerability, writes that women are taught to be quiet, and, if they do otherwise, they often feel shame. The following are the kinds of messages women shared with her, messages that got in the way of their authentic expression:

- ▸ Don't make people feel uncomfortable but be honest.
- ▸ Don't upset anyone or hurt anyone's feelings but say what's on your mind.
- ▸ Sound informed and educated but not like a know-it-all.
- ▸ Don't say anything unpopular or controversial but have the courage to disagree with the crowd.[5]

---

5   Brown, *The Gifts of Imperfection*, 52.

Each of these messages is a perfect example of a contra-diction that may make you feel like you're going crazy. And this research wasn't even specifically about speaking out in the *sexual* realm.

In the United States, we have much to be grateful for regarding our freedoms of expression, dress, and careers as women. If you talk to a woman who was born as recently as the early 1940s and ask if she had the same free-doms growing up, you'll hear about some drastic changes around finances, marriage, and birth control. These advancements in gender equality and social consciousness are profound and important. Nonetheless, discrimination still exists based on gender, sexual orientation, continuing racial prejudices, and some archaic sexual beliefs.

Let's begin with our collective discomfort with sex. Many politicians and religious leaders desperately want to "protect our children" from frank, open conversations about what it means to be a healthy sexual being—as if even hearing about sex will corrupt innocent children. But even in more progressive segments of society in which adults recognize the positive aspects of sexuality, a joyous and balanced approach to sex education rarely makes it into conversations with adolescents. A danger-prevention and risk-management approach is the norm.[6] This does not protect children; it means that they are ill-equipped to understand the complexity of sexual interactions. And our society's consistently negative messaging—don't get preg-nant, sex is dangerous, don't have sex before marriage—is often instilled in girls more than in boys.

---

6   Deborah L. Tolman and Sara I. McClelland, "Normative Sexuality Development in Adolescence: A Decade in Review, 2000–2009," *Journal of Research on Adolescence* 21, no. 1 (2011): 242–255.

There are also many contradictions in the messages young women hear: Women are not as sexual as men, but in rape situations, they really wanted it. Women should not be "too" sexual, but they should please their partners and be passionate in bed. Plus, there is still a heavy "good girl" ideology that teaches many young women to be quiet, feminine, nice, and obedient—to put the needs of others first, even to their own detriment. In my opinion, the good girl ideology—this expectation of quiet femininity imposed on girls—is the foundation of Brené Brown's findings about shame and our fear of speaking out.

In our society, the traits instilled in women are valued less than those instilled in men. The concerns of women are taken less seriously as well, and their voices dismissed or ignored. An example of the terrible consequence of the confluence of these factors is the ability of someone like Larry Nasser, a doctor for the American gymnastics team, to sexually abuse hundreds of girls over many years. He was able to abuse his power as a male doctor, in part because most of the "obedient" and "nice" girls he abused were not empowered to question his behavior, and those who spoke up had their accusations brushed under the rug.

One definition of madness is "extremely foolish behavior."[7] Even a cursory examination of our cultural expectations and messages around female sexuality will point to their absurdities and contradictions. From a sociological perspective, such messages can create in women an unhealthy relationship with their bodies,

7   *English Oxford Living Dictionaries*, s.v. "madness," accessed July 9, 2013, en.oxforddictionaries.com/definition/madness.

minds, identities, and sexuality. The madness is that girls are taught—through parents and religion, classroom sex education, advertising, the mass media, and even some governmental information—to dislike their bodies, to be ashamed of their desires, or to compare themselves to a male version of sexuality. Then, as adult women in long-term, loving relationships, they are expected—as if by magic—to be free and open with their sexuality, to explore their authentic selves, to connect deeply with their partner, and to easily give and receive pleasure. And this passionate attitude is supposed to last the life of a long-term relationship. Those expectations, however, rarely meet reality.

Very few people can suddenly flip a switch to love their bodies and love themselves as fully expressed sexual beings. The field of social neuroscience shows how habits, beliefs, and negative emotions create deep and efficient patterns of behavior in our brain. This points to the importance of deprogramming *and* reprogramming the brain, and those both take time.[8] The fact that our brains possess the quality of neuroplasticity, meaning we actually *can* program, deprogram, and reprogram our minds, is amazing in itself. Mindfulness practices are a powerful way to access this neuroplasticity, to change habits and patterns, even when they are well-worn grooves. It takes time, but it can be done. But before we understand *how* to change these patterns, I want to explore *what* these patterns of beliefs might be for you, and where you may

---

8   If neuropsychology and neuroscience interest you in the realm of personal growth, I really enjoyed the book *Buddha's Brain: The Practical Neuroscience of Happiness, Love, and Wisdom*, by Rick Hanson, PhD.

have learned them. Knowing that what you've been taught is not necessarily natural or normal, and that you are not alone in having learned these potentially destructive habits, can liberate you. I hope you're already starting to feel the juice!

A common definition of insanity, actually based on the findings of Sigmund Freud, is doing the same thing over and over again, but expecting different results. I rather like this definition, and I ask you to consider: If things aren't working for you sexually, perhaps it is time to try something truly different? If not, you will likely be stuck in the same patterns for a long time, even a lifetime. I would be remiss if I didn't also mention "hysteria," a nineteenth-century term for madness that reflects the way we've labeled and judged women for thousands of years.[9] *Hysteria* was a catch-all term used to explain a variety of women's symptoms, such as anxiety, irritation, weakness, or even sexual desire. "Hyster" refers to the uterus (as in the word *hysterectomy*), which was considered a medical reason why women were the weaker sex and also more prone to madness. You know—clearly the little ladies needed men to take care of them, because they were too weak or unstable to take care of themselves. Even today, a woman who publicly displays too much emotion—particularly anger—may be labeled "hysterical" as a way of trivializing her and portraying her views as irrational or unreliable. Such labels were madness then, and are madness now.

Think about the hottest topics in sex in our society. Pornography? Virginity? Orgasm? Consent? Rape? All

---

9   Cecilia Tasca, "Women and Hysteria in the History of Mental Health," *Clinical Practice & Epidemiology in Mental Health* 8, no. 1 (2012): 110–119.

of these areas and more have great significance for a woman's sexual experiences. In the following sections, I am going to paint a picture, based on research and my experiences from more than twenty years in the field, to show you what's going on culturally today and what we've been taught about female sexuality. Perhaps some details of this picture won't resonate with you, but I'm guessing that, if you chose to pick up this book, many will—for you as well as your sisters, daughters, mothers, and friends. Demographic factors also weave together in the complex tapestry of an individual woman's sexual experiences; these factors include race and ethnicity, sexual orientation, education level, religious upbringing and affiliation, age, parental status, and relationship status or form.

I invite you to reflect, as you read these sections, on whether and how all of these demographic factors have impacted your development as a sexual woman. This is a heavy chapter. My fellow sociologists and I joke that sociologists are professional buzzkills. If you're curious about the detailed ways our societal training creates shame and confusion around female sexuality, you'll love this chapter. If not, feel free to skim and move on. But I do promise you, this book overall is about hope.

WHAT THE RESEARCH SAYS

Imagine you are a fifteen-year-old girl in American society today. You got your first period at age twelve, but you didn't receive much education about it except some silly cartoons from an uncomfortable gym teacher who had to teach health class. You feel embarrassed that your body is going through these changes, and you've only heard negative things about periods. You notice that your continually changing body is something that gets attention from boys at school. You're still not sure how you feel about boys at this point, and you feel self-conscious about the attention. But you also like some of the attention, and you think it means that the boys like you and that you're pretty. For as long as you can remember, adults have commented when they thought you looked nice, and this attention made you feel good and taught you that your looks are important. You kind of have a crush on one of the boys in your math class, and wonder what it will be like to fall in love and how you'll know. You start posting photos on Instagram and create Snapchat videos, making sure the camera angles show your growing cleavage in flattering ways. You mimic shots you've seen on other Instagram feeds, and you get more attention at school. But one day someone writes "SLUT!" online, under one of your photos. Someone else, thinking she is funny, writes about how you've slept with all the guys in your class in high school. Just like that, your life is a living hell. That's all it takes.

This is what can happen when girls are taught that their value is in their appearance and sex appeal, but at the same time, "slut-shaming" and the derogation of the female body is a huge part of their culture. This is one of the many unfortunate dangers of social media's impact on girls. The slut stigma has been around for a long time, but now it has a way to spread—whether based on actual sexual behavior or not—in a day. Couple this with young women learning that the number of likes and positive comments on their social media posts is indicative of their attractiveness and sexiness, and you see how they become trapped in a dangerous cycle. The stigma of "slut" has a very real impact on young women's lives and has even had the unfortunate outcome of suicide for some young women.[10]

There's no doubt that as humans, women and men have more similarities than differences. However, from birth, girls and boys are treated differently, based on assumptions about what it means to be feminine versus masculine and on the assumption that everyone should fit into one of those categories. Although being unique and nonconformist may be cool, most people follow relatively strict rules about what is appropriate for their gender. This is understandable because in most circles, being a gender nonconformist is considered weird and deserving of ridicule and shaming (although living in San Diego, I see this changing in some of our local high schools, as teenagers who break from the traditional gender binary gain acceptance and support).

Regarding gender expectations for women specifically, research has found that the qualities most desired in women include being thin, modest, and nice.[11] These traits require self-control and suppressing one's voice while prioritizing the needs of others. If this is what most women think they need to be, and what most partners or business settings expect of them, it is no surprise we have a cadre of women playing small ball in their lives overall and in their sex lives specifically. Traditional gender-role socialization for women does not encourage

10   Lewis M. Webb, "Shame Transfigured: Slut-Shaming from Rome to Cyberspace," *First Monday* 20, no. 4 (2015). doi: http://dx.doi.org/10.5210/fm.v20i4.5464

11   James R. Mahalik et al., "Development of the Conformity to Feminine Norms Inventory," *Sex Roles* 52, nos. 7–8 (2005): 417–435.

them to know themselves, like themselves, and feel confident in speaking up for their thoughts and needs. Women of color, and young women who find themselves attracted to other women, can face even greater backlash when speaking up for themselves.

Women are often perceived negatively when they talk openly about their sexuality and take ownership of their pleasure, and the situation mentioned previously is a common example of how shame is used to police female sexuality. Being perceived as "too sexual," even if their sexuality exists only in the gossip of others, is a slippery slope for females, and that perception impacts how they are treated, regarded, talked about, etc.[12] Many young women are taught to protect and project an image of themselves as "good girls," or at least not to project whatever is considered promiscuous. Men on the other hand, often gain status by having many sex partners or casual sexual relationships.[13]

While men overall are granted greater sexual expression than women, theirs is limited in its own way by societal expectations of masculinity. For example, Brené Brown writes about the difficulty and fear men have in ever appearing weak.[14] Yet weakness, or more accurately, vulnerability, is necessary to maintain a healthy and communicative long-term relationship and sex life. A fantastic documentary

---

12   Eric S. Blumberg, "The Lives and Voices of Highly Sexual Women," *Journal of Sex Research* 40, no. 2 (2003): 146–157.

13   Laurie A. Rudman, Janell C. Fetterolf, and Diana T. Sanchez, "What Motivates the Sexual Double Standard? More Support for Male Versus Female Control Theory," *Personality and Social Psychology Bulletin* 39, no. 2 (2013): 250–263.

14   Brené Brown, *Daring Greatly: How the Courage to Be Vulnerable Transforms the Way We Live, Love, Parent, and Lead* (New York: Gotham Books, 2012).

about the negative impact of traditional masculinity on men, *The Mask You Live In*, shows how our messaging around masculinity creates young men who struggle with authenticity. They are shamed out of feeling and expressing the full range of their human emotions and don't have safe spaces (especially with other men) to be messy and real. The weight of this version of masculinity can be heavier for men in some subcultures, such as those raised around the military, in African American and Latino cultures, and in some working-class neighborhoods. The social norms of gender role expectations can work against all of us.

The "good girl" ideology imposed on many females versus the "boys will be boys" mentality for males has a large impact on our sexuality. These socially desirable behaviors are reflected in the ways women and men respond on sexual surveys—unless they think they are attached to a lie detector. Psychology professor and researcher Terri Fisher found that college students will misrepresent the number of sexual partners they have had (more for men and less for women) unless they believe they are being monitored by a lie detector device. The most interesting part of her research is that students didn't lie when it came to other gendered activities in which they were breaking social norms (e.g., women using obscene language or men writing poetry). Fisher concluded that sexuality is unique among other activities, with expected gender differences exerting a strong pull and a greater desire to fit in, even in one's own mind.[15] No wonder so many women have an odd relationship with sex!

15   Terri D. Fisher, "Gender Roles and Pressure to Be Truthful: The Bogus Pipeline Modifies Gender Differences in Sexual but Not Non-Sexual Behavior," *Sex Roles* 68, nos. 7–8 (2013): 401–414.

Now I'm going to take you on a brief (and fascinating) tour of recent research into some of the biggest topics around female sexuality, and I will also share my own thoughts, as a sociologist and sexologist, about what's going on. While there is much more to each of these specific topics than I can cover in this book, I hope to give you enough information to see how the madness surfaces in all aspects of how we're taught to behave sexually as females. Again, you may discover that if you have struggled in any of these areas, you are not alone.

Masturbation and Fantasies

Many of us don't have a good picture of what women actually do when they masturbate. This might seem like a minor thing, but it becomes less so when you consider that understanding masturbation means you understand the basic ways women achieve sexual pleasure and satisfaction. A study of undergraduate women found that those who masturbated were more likely to have accurate knowledge of the clitoris.[16] Our general lack of information about female pleasure has been revealed in recent years thanks to the influx of quality sex toys designed for women's bodies. Motivated by the desire to sell products, companies creating and selling such sex toys have needed to conduct research to better understand how women masturbate. Still, the general population tends to make inaccurate assumptions about female self-pleasure. This is perhaps because we base our understanding of sexuality on male sexuality. As a group, men

---

16   Lisa Wade, Emily Kremer, and Jessica Brown, "The Incidental Orgasm: The Presence of Clitoral Knowledge and the Absence of Orgasm for Women," *Women & Health* 42, no. 1 (2005): 117–138.

tend to masturbate in very similar ways, by manually gripping their penises. Women, on the other hand, have a much greater range in their masturbatory styles and tempos, and legendary sex researchers Masters and Johnson found that no two women masturbated exactly the same way.[17] Nonetheless, one qualitative research study found that women assumed most other women masturbated by penetrating their vaginas, despite evidence to the contrary.[18]

In my own interviews with thirty-five women about their sexual experiences, the question, "How do you masturbate?" was fraught with discomfort. Across the board, these women eventually gave detailed accounts of how they touch themselves and the progression of their touch, although it was clear that none had ever discussed this before. Positions ranged from lying on one's belly with a vibrator between a pillow and the clitoris, to lying on one's back with legs tightly together and rocking while touching the vulva, to a seated position with legs pulled in. Methods included using a vibrator or just one's fingers, using lubricant or not. They mentioned a variety of vibrators and toys for clitoral stimulation, vaginal penetration, and anal play. The possibilities seem truly endless!

As indicated by their social discomfort, many women are aware of the contradiction between the private plea-

---

17   William H. Masters and Virginia E. Johnson, *Human Sexual Response* (Boston: Little, Brown & Co, 1966).

18   Breanne Fahs and Elena Frank, "Notes from the Back Room: Gender, Power, and (In)Visibility in Women's Experiences of Masturbation," *The Journal of Sex Research* 51, no. 3 (2013): 241–252.

sure of masturbation and the social stigma,[19] the same stigma that leads to embarrassment or shame. Yet the cultural and often religion-based shame regarding masturbation, especially for females, is quite odd when you step back and examine it. Self-pleasure is truly a private activity that does no harm and makes people happy.[20] According to a national study in 2010, more than 50 percent of the women surveyed, ages eighteen to forty-nine, had masturbated at some point in the previous ninety days.[21] Nonetheless, even though scientific research has found that the encouragement of masturbation would be a smart strategy to prevent the spread of STDs and STIs (sexually transmitted infections), avoid unwanted pregnancies, and improve sexual health awareness and intimacy within relationships, many mainstream leaders in scientific and educational fields will not recommend the practice.[22] Apparently it does not matter that masturbation has so many positive aspects when decisions are based on uncomfortable emotions and sexual taboos.

---

19   Christine Elizabeth Kaestle and Katherine R. Allen, "The Role of Masturbation in Healthy Sexual Development: Perceptions of Young Adults," *Archives of Sexual Behavior* 40, no. 5 (2011): 983–994.

20   I'm not talking here about the small number of people who end up in the emergency room at 2 a.m. with objects stuck in their rectums, nor folks who masturbate to the exclusion of other life priorities.

21   Debby Herbenick, Michael Reece, Vanessa Schick, Stephanie A. Sanders, Brian Dodge, and J. Dennis Fortenberry. "Sexual Behaviors, Relationships, and Perceived Health Status Among Adult Women in the United States: Results from a National Probability Sample." *The Journal of Sexual Medicine* 7 (2010): 277-290.

22   Kaestle and Allen, "The Role of Masturbation in Healthy Sexual Development," 983–994.

The first-ever documentary on masturbation, called *Sticky: A (Self) Love Story*, was released in 2016. This thought-provoking, educational, and entertaining documentary chronicles our social, medical, political, and religious views on this sticky topic. I was one of the experts interviewed for the movie back in 2008, but unfortunately, it took the producers many years to complete the film because they ran into so many roadblocks. Societal discomfort around the topic is so high that funders and potential assistants literally didn't want to touch it.[23]

Another area in which women tend to feel shame and fear judgment is around their sexual fantasies. Women sometimes judge themselves for the content of their own fantasies, thinking there is something wrong about these imaginings. In my private practice, I often need to help women normalize their enjoyment of fantasy, teaching them that sexual fantasies are natural and also that the content of such fantasies is fine. One of the more common fantasies women have is being forced, dominated, or controlled sexually.[24] Since it is so common, I want to mention it here, both to normalize it and to point out that just because a woman fantasizes about being forced sexually does not mean that she really wants it to happen. Even if she enjoys being with a dominant sexual partner, that sexual interaction is still within a safe and consensual environment. I want to make this point because I think that sometimes women are embarrassed about this specific fantasy: They

---

23   If you'd like to learn more about *Sticky: A (Self) Love Story*, visit the documentary website at www.stickythemovie.com

24   Donald S. Strassberg and Lisa K. Locker, "Force in Women's Sexual Fantasies," *Archives of Sex Behavior* 27, no. 4 (1998): 403–414, doi:10.1023/A:1018740210472.

think it means they must really want such forced encounters to happen. So I'm here to set the record straight: No, it does not mean that you really want it to happen. But maybe you do want that kind of dominant energy in a sexual interaction, and if you want to consensually negotiate that sexual scenario with a partner, that's just fine, too.

Virginity and Avoiding Pregnancy

In our society, females and virginity also have an odd relationship. Virginity is often—particularly within religious contexts—still discussed as a "gift" that a woman gives to a man. Or it's addressed as something that the female needs to protect, because once she has given it away, she'll never be pure again. An extreme example of this can be seen in the Elizabeth Smart abduction case. She was kidnapped from her Salt Lake City home in 2002 at the age of fourteen. She was held captive for nine months and raped daily until she was rescued. Growing up, she learned through her religion that sex should be saved for marriage, and that if a girl had sex, she was like a "chewed-up piece of gum" that no one would want. And so, although Smart had opportunities to escape, one of the reasons she did not was because she felt dirty and unworthy. The loss of her "purity" was the loss of her self-worth.[25]

Our traditional understanding of virginity is what sociologists call *heteronormative*, meaning that it's based on the assumption that everyone is or should be heterosexual, and ascribes to the traditional view of biological sex and gender as binary, only male or female. The

---

25   Elizabeth Smart shared this story at Johns Hopkins Bloomberg School of Public Health; the video is available on YouTube: youtu.be/kzBVzBf-Dn4

heteronormative view of virginity is that it is "lost" when a penis enters a vagina. But if the definition of losing one's virginity, for a female, is having one's vagina penetrated by a penis, does this mean that a lesbian who is only ever with women never loses her virginity?[26] Likewise, if a woman engages in oral or anal sex with a partner of any gender identity, has she lost her virginity? Or, for a girl who is unfortunately molested as a child, does that mean that she is not a virgin?

Interestingly, in a small study of teenagers about the "loss" of their virginity, almost one-third of the participants did not think that rape counted as a loss of virginity. This means that not only is the specific sexual act relevant to some teens, but factors such as consent are, too.[27] This topic of virginity makes me recall confusing conversations in graduate school with friends from Middle Eastern countries about their definition of virginity. Their definition was centered around sexual activity overall, and not just penile penetration. Without cultural comparisons such as these, we may fall into the trap of assuming that the sexual definitions and norms we grow up with are the "natural" or only norms. I assure you, they are not.

Virginity is incredibly ambiguous, which is a good indicator that the definition is not scientific. It is an attempt,

26   Paige Averett, Amy Moore, and Lindsay Price, "Virginity Definitions and Meaning among the LGBT Community," *Journal of Gay & Lesbian Social Services* 26, no. 3 (2014): 259–278, doi:10.1080/10538720.2014.924802 I found it insightful to read that the coming-out process can be much more of a rite of passage for LGBT youth than the loss of virginity.

27   Jeremy E. Uecker, Nicole Angotti, and Mark D. Regnerus, "Going Most of the Way: 'Technical Virginity' among American Adolescents," *Social Science Research* 37, no. 4 (2008): 1200–1215.

mostly moral and cultural, at controlling female sexuality, and likely has a foundation in the practice of only passing ownership of land on to a man's biological heirs. This means that the societal and religious concerns about female virginity are really based in men's need to ensure their children are genetic heirs for their inheritances. There are many other directions I could take this analysis of virginity, but if there's any conclusion to be drawn from research on this topic, it's that virginity has many socially constructed components and creates a weight of judgment and fear for many young women.

Prior to reliable birth control methods such as the hormonal pill, virginity was also emphasized to avoid out-of-wedlock pregnancy. However, even now, there are religious groups and political leaders who discourage the use of contraception and believe it is sinful because they claim it goes against the will of God. For women whose belief system, whether religious, cultural, or political, inhibits the use of birth control, virginity is still touted as the best way to avoid unwanted pregnancies. And as such, there are still harsh criticisms of young women who fail to uphold the expectations of abstinence and virginity until marriage.

It's also fascinating that for many years there has been talk of a hormonal birth control pill for men that is "just around the corner." But lack of funding, combined with the drug's tested side effects impacting men's sexuality (side effects that are similar to what women experience on the pill), continually halts the progress of this research. Clearly the responsibility for preventing pregnancy is still placed on a woman's shoulders.

Period Embarrassment

Anxiety, shame, misinformation, and even disgust permeate conversations around our periods. Sure, menstruation is not the most pleasant experience, but our levels of emotional embarrassment and revulsion go far beyond any physical discomfort and are largely learned in childhood. Have you ever boldly and openly carried a tampon as you walked to a restroom? The fact that I even use the word "boldly" reveals that this would take courage. Many of us are ill-prepared for our first periods. And if we do know much about it, our reaction is likely to be negative, or even frightened. A small study of eighteen- to twenty-one-year-old women found that all of the participants still carried some kind of discomfort, embarrassment, and body shame from their initial menstrual experience. Early experiences—such as the embarrassment and confusion I experienced in fourth grade—continue to frame menstrual experiences as women age.[28]

Culturally, we are taught that all aspects of periods should be kept hidden. That certainly doesn't engender a feeling of comfort around a monthly process that couldn't be more natural. I remember having a serious boyfriend when I was in my mid-thirties who reacted with disgust when I had a few tampons sitting on the back of the toilet for easy access in the middle of the night. They were unused and wrapped. But he still openly expressed disgust, and was self-righteous in doing so, without awareness of the potential shaming impact on me. Thankfully, I had the confidence to just tell him to grow up. If I hadn't been in

---

28   Theresa E. Jackson and Rachel Joffe Falmagne, "Women Wearing White: Discourses of Menstruation and the Experience of Menarche," *Feminism & Psychology* 23, no. 3 (2013): 379–398.

my thirties and already in the sexual health field, it would have been more difficult not to internalize that shame or embarrassment.

What about sex during menstruation? This can be seen as taboo to discuss and distasteful to practice. One research study found that the majority of women had negative reactions to this idea, but that most of their negativity came from trying to avoid their partner's discomfort or disgust. White women and women who identified as bisexual or lesbian were more likely to report positive emotions around sexual play during menstruation, compared to women of color and heterosexual women.[29] While we might have some of our own personal reactions to our blood and menstrual discharge, these reactions also carry a very strong, negative, and culturally learned component worth examining.

And what happens when a woman moves through menopause and stops having periods? Many people don't really know, because we don't talk openly about this as a society! There is shame and silence from the beginning through the end of our menstrual years. While each woman's actual experience of going through this phase of life is individually varied, societal attitudes toward menopause tend towards the negative. If you haven't yet experienced menopause, what are your thoughts about it? It's likely that you imagine a negative experience you are not looking forward to. Maybe menopause to you signals that you will no longer be attractive, or be a woman in the same way, or that you won't ever be sexual

29   Breanne Fahs, "Sex During Menstruation: Race, Sexual Identity, and Women's Accounts of Pleasure and Disgust," *Feminism & Psychology* 21, no. 2 (2011): 155–178.

again. Maybe you fear it will be a period of uncomfortable and unpleasant bodily changes, such as temperature fluctuations, vaginal dryness, and weight gain, or unpredictable emotional changes. Although women can experience many physical and emotional changes, none of these outcomes are necessarily true for all women. A meta-analysis of studies on attitudes toward menopause and the subsequent experience of menopause found that women who had negative expectations were indeed more likely to have negative experiences during menopause![30] As I'll discuss in future chapters, our expectations can create our reality.

Lack of Real Sex Education

What did you learn about your body, your menstrual cycle, or the functioning of your sexual anatomy in school? Depending on where you lived, you might have received little sex education, and, in particular, you probably heard very little about female sexual pleasure. As a late bloomer, I didn't start dating until my senior year of high school, and I learned about the existence of my clitoris from my first boyfriend (and I'm lucky *he* knew about it!). I think it's ridiculous that I had to learn about a sexual body part from a man who doesn't even have the same anatomy. This is not the way to empower young women about their bodies and their own pleasure.

Women's stories about their orgasms repeatedly show that the clitoris is at the heart of the female orgasm.

---

30   Beverley Ayers, Mark Forshaw, and Myra S. Hunter, "The Impact of Attitudes toward Menopause on Women's Symptom Experience: A Systematic Review," *Maturitas* 65, no. 1 (2010): 28–36, doi:10.1016/j.maturitas.2009.10.016.

Nonetheless, each generation continues to be indoc-
trinated into the myth that women can orgasm reliably
through penetrative intercourse. Years ago I was teaching
a female sexual empowerment and sex toy workshop for
women, and stated that only about 25 percent of women
can reliably orgasm through penetrative intercourse
without some kind of direct clitoral stimulation. One of
the workshop participants asked if I would call her fiancé
and repeat that information. Despite her explanation that
such orgasms during intercourse were not common for
women, he still believed that there was something wrong
with *her* and her inability to orgasm. Unfortunately, I
didn't see her again, so I don't know if her fiancé was
willing to learn about and appreciate her unique sexual
functioning . . . or whether she still married him!

What is the impact of this overall lack of comprehensive sex education on women's sexual health? Well, in
the United States each year, more than 750,000 young
women (aged fifteen to nineteen) become pregnant, and
at least 80 percent of these pregnancies are unintended.[31]
Imagine, though, if young women were taught to know
their bodies and that they have the right to their own pleasure and the right to have boundaries with others—and
that sexual activity can be both amazing and crushing?
And then imagine that they were taught what to do with
all of this complexity, and how to make the healthiest
long-term decisions for their own well-being? Clearly this
isn't the norm, so many young women don't know how
to avoid dangers like STDs/STIs; indeed, for fifteen- to

---

31   Lorrie Gavin et al., "Sexual and Reproductive Health of
Persons Aged 10–24 Years—United States, 2002–2007," *Surveillance
Summaries* 58, no. SS-6 (2009).

nineteen-year-old women, the Centers for Disease Control and Prevention estimates that one in four has an STI.[32] With statistics this blatant, plus the clear impact that ignorance has on female sexual satisfaction, how can we keep making the decision to "protect" our teen girls by *not* talking about sex?

I want to add to this section on poor sex education that we also have a lack of *relationship* education. Did you ever have a class in high school where you learned how to recognize your emotions and needs and then responsibly articulate them to another? The Hollywood romantic version of relationships portrays love as easy. But it takes emotional intelligence skills and negotiation skills, within a foundation of mindful awareness and compassion, to develop a healthy relationship. Part of navigating a successful relationship is knowing that there is no "perfect" relationship that meets all your needs without conflict. Relationships also involve working together as a team through everyday activities, arguments, and goals.[33] In chapter 3 I delve into common obstacles to healthy relationships and communication, with many exercises to help you learn the skills never taught in school.

---

32   Hillard Weinstock, Stuart Berman, and Willard Cates, Jr., "Sexually Transmitted Diseases among American Youth: Incidence and Prevalence Estimates, 2000," *Perspectives on Sexual and Reproductive Health* 36, no. 1 (2004): 6–10.

33   I really love John Gottman's research and work on creating happy relationships. I think his book *The Seven Principles for Making Marriage Work* is an invaluable resource in any relationship.

Sexual Activities

If talking to teen girls about vaginal intercourse is taboo, topics like anal sex are even more so. But that doesn't mean this activity isn't happening. A study of Latina and black teenagers found that approximately one-third had engaged in heterosexual anal intercourse, and most of them did not use a condom.[34] If you haven't brushed up on your HIV 101 recently, I'll remind you that anal sex has a higher transmission rate for HIV, primarily because the anus has more fragile tissue and does not self-lubricate like the vagina. Small tears are more likely to occur, thereby exposing the body to more risk of infection. What tends to happen, though, is that our societal and personal discomfort with sexual topics is also socialized into our health-care workers. And these folks, like most folks, are uncomfortable with discussions about certain kinds of sexual activities. This means that they are not able to adequately address these nitty-gritty sexual topics with adolescents who desperately need the education. Hence, the madness cycle continues.

An interesting question to consider is whether these young women, and adult women for that matter, *want* to engage in anal sex. Please know that I am not intending to denigrate anal sex or those who desire it—the anus has many nerve endings, the stimulation of which can bring great pleasure for women, sometimes even facilitating orgasm. The piece that's most relevant to this chapter, though, is that many females may be reluctantly pushed

---

34   Carol F. Roye, Beatrice J. Krauss, and Paula L. Silverman, "Prevalence and Correlates of Heterosexual Anal Intercourse among Black and Latina Female Adolescents," *Journal of the Association of Nurses in AIDS Care* 21, no. 4 (2010): 291–301.

into trying anal activity by males, or might choose it as a way to maintain their "technical" virginity. And while it has great potential for pleasure, it can also have great potential for pain, bleeding, and discomfort if the participants don't know what they're doing. A fascinating small qualitative study delved into this topic and found that all of the women interviewed who had engaged, or tried to engage, in anal sex with their male partner were motivated by wanting to please their partner—prioritizing emotional connection over physical pain, or hoping to seem "normal." And sometimes the women's acquiescence was just blatant coercion by their partner.[35] Clearly there's a lot going on around the back door, and we're not comfortable talking about it.

Oral sex has become more of a sexual norm for younger generations, particularly for girls performing oral sex on boys. In the documentary *Oral Sex Is the New Goodnight Kiss*, teen girls performing oral sex on teen boys is shown as a normal part of teen activity and a path to social status and power. (This documentary primarily delves into teen girls trading sexual favors for status and clothing, then getting recruited into teen prostitution by other teen girls in Canada's affluent suburbs.)[36] Two points are worth highlighting here. One is that female sexual performance is seen as social currency. A quick

---

35 Breanne Fahs and Jax Gonzalez, "The Front Lines of the 'Back Door': Navigating (Dis)engagement, Coercion, and Pleasure in Women's Anal Sex Experiences," *Feminism & Psychology* 24, no. 4 (2014): 500–520.

36 Learn more about the documentary and book at https://www.goodreads.com/book/show/6746357-oral-sex-is-the-new-goodnight-kiss

look at our national media and advertising, plastered with images of the female body, explains where young women are learning this.

The second point is the question of whether female sexual pleasure is involved in such exchanges. Are these girls receiving the pleasure of oral sex in return, or, more generally, are their male partners also prioritizing female sexual pleasure? Based on research by Peggy Orenstein in her fantastic book *Girls & Sex*, this is not the case.[37] Equality in giving and receiving pleasure is highly relevant to gendered sexual experiences but largely absent from our sex education dialogues. Since we rarely teach teen girls that sexual activities can and should feel good, and that they have a right to that pleasure, it becomes normalized that their sexual performance is in the service of pleasure for others.

Women's Pleasure and Orgasm

For some women, receiving sexual pleasure makes them feel vulnerable. Being present in the moment and willing to surrender to the potential release and abandon of orgasm can make them feel too raw or out of control, or self-conscious about *how* they orgasm. Women tend to take longer than men to reach orgasm, and again, since much of what we learn about sexuality is through the lens of male sexual experience, a quicker orgasm in every sexual encounter is considered the norm. A young female client shared with me that she was embarrassed that she took so long to reach orgasm with her partner. When I

---

37 I can't recommend this book enough if you're interested in understanding how girls are trying to navigate the complicated sexual landscape in American society today.

asked her how long it generally took, she said about five
to ten minutes. I gently informed her that some women
can take forty-five minutes, so she was not on the far side
of that continuum. When you combine lack of knowledge
about how women like to be pleased with an unfounded
expectation of easy, quick orgasms, it's not surprising that
faking orgasm is so common. A British study of sexually active heterosexual college women reported that 80
percent of the women indicated they had faked orgasms in
half of their sexual interactions.[38] Half! Yikes.

When our expectations surrounding sex come from a
male perspective, women understandably fall embarrass-
ingly short of those measures. A sexual encounter is often
considered "over" when the male has an orgasm. A penis
defines virginity, and a penis defines a sexual encounter.
I'm not saying that all men or all sexual encounters are
like this; what I am saying is that these beliefs have long
shaped our culture's sexual landscape.

The authors of an article on "Mindfulness and Good
Enough Sex" explain how many women really operate: "A
more typical pattern is to be orgasmic in approximately
70 percent of sexual encounters using multiple stimulation before and during intercourse. Another common
pattern is to be orgasmic during erotic, non-intercourse
sex (i.e., manual, oral, rubbing or vibrator stimulation)
and seldom, if at all, during intercourse."[39] Again, while

---

38   Gayle Brewer and Colin A. Hendrie, "Evidence to Suggest that
Copulatory Vocalizations in Women Are Not a Reflexive Consequence
of Orgasm," *Archives of Sexual Behavior* 40, no. 3 (2010): 559–564.

39   Barry McCarthy and Lana M. Wald, "Mindfulness and Good
Enough Sex," *Sexual and Relationship Therapy* 28, nos. 1–2 (2013):
39–47.

women and men have many more similarities than differences, the differences can be impactful and significant when they aren't acknowledged.

Pornography

Pornography plays an interesting role in our society. When I talk about pornography, I'm referencing the statistically most prevalent and mainstream versions of porn, designed by and for heterosexual men. Pornography is supposed to be about sexual openness, expression, and pleasure, but most of it is created for the specific viewing pleasure of heterosexual males. Given that porn is rarely an accurate portrayal of safe and consensual sexual practices, it is unfortunate that in the absence of effective sex education, pornography accounts for so much of the sex and gender role education of our youth and adults. And few adults have discussions with their teens about the values being espoused.[40] Activities depicted in mainstream, easily accessible pornography often become popular as mainstream sexual practices within ten years. This may account for the increasing migration of anal sex practices from porn contexts to real-life contexts. Pornography now plays a big role in shaping our sexual landscape, beliefs, desires, and actions.

This shift may be connected to a more obvious change in cultural beliefs about the "sexually liberated female." Over the last few decades, it became cool for young women to let young men know that they were free with showing their bodies, going to strip clubs, or

---

40   Kath Albury, "Porn and Sex Education, Porn as Sex Education," *Porn Studies* 1, nos. 1–2 (2014): 172–181.

watching pornography. It has become a badge of honor for some young women to show that they are cooler than other girls because they aren't offended by such things. But does that actually mean that they are sexually liberated?

Sometimes young women do what I call "performing porn star." This is when women act in sexual ways that they think are expected of them because of what they've seen in porn videos. While in and of itself this doesn't have to be a bad thing, the role has two problematic aspects: First, a woman who sexually performs is likely limiting herself in her sexual expression to what she thinks is appropriate and expected; and second, she is objectifying herself instead of being interested in her own pleasure. This means that she emphasizes performing and pleasing her partner, rather than feeling her own embodied sensations and pleasure. This is another reason why women fake orgasms—it's hard to reach orgasm when you're not connected to your own pleasurable sensations.

Mainstream pornography portrays "lesbians"—which really means "girl-on-girl action"—primarily for the pleasure of men. Women are often depicted sexually interacting with other women primarily for the pleasure of the men in the video who are watching, and for the home viewing audience. This representation is quite different from the real experience of women who are sexually and emotionally attracted to other women for their own fulfillment and that of their partner. Yet this pornographic version of "lesbianism" seems to be pervasive in heterosexual men's fantasies and their understandings of lesbians. Although such a representation may play out positively in a greater acceptance of sexual fluidity for women in the United States, it is also offensive and trivializing of genuine and loving interactions between women.

Because pornography is made primarily for hetero-sexual men's pleasure, the women are often depicted as a version of a male fantasy. And because some women feel the expectation to live up to and perform what they see in porn, they also may start to hold themselves to the unreasonable standards of fantasy. Much of mainstream porn focuses on thin women with large (often fake) breasts, hairless vulvas, and full makeup who like to be dominated and have quick and easy orgasms. If women take these images as the standard for their sexual expres-sion, they are setting themselves up for self-criticism and detachment from their own pleasure.

Our Rape Culture and Culture of Coercion

What is "rape culture" and how is that term relevant here? The term itself describes prevailing social norms around gender, sex, and communication that lead to an implicit normalizing of sexual assault, blaming women, and enjoying humor about rape. In a rape culture, sexual coercion becomes a normal part of sexual interaction.[41] While this might sound extreme, consider the facts about one of our nationally publicized high school rape cases, where there was social media footage of a group of athletes sexually assaulting a high school girl: There were many witnesses, but no one stopped the rape; it was difficult to get witnesses to come forward, and the athletes' coaches

---

41   While the term "rape culture" is often used, I prefer the terms "coercion culture" and its opposite, "consent culture." They receive a less divisive reaction and allow us all more space to change and grow.

joked about what had happened and tried to conceal it.[42] These facts are alarming and compelling. Unfortunately, they represent a common response in publicized rape cases, especially in colleges and universities.

I think it's most helpful to consider the underlying assumptions that facilitate such responses to a rape, such as: the girl really wants it, asking for consent is unnecessary, unwanted sexual activity is not that serious, taking what you want sexually is something to be joked about, and protecting men from the harm of being charged with sexual assault is much more important than seeking justice for the harm done to the young woman. These prevailing attitudes result from a basic misunderstanding about female sexual pleasure and desire—the assumption that if a man is enjoying the sexual encounter, then the person he's with likely is as well. These prevailing attitudes also result from an unspoken belief that the young woman's voice, needs, and feelings don't matter as much as those of the young man. The negative impact on her matters less than any impact on him. If this isn't an example of ingrained sexism, I don't know what is.

As an aside, I know that some women claim rape after a night of sexual activity that they wished hadn't happen, or to get revenge on a partner or a man who hurt them. Yes, that does happen. Is it statistically the norm? *No. Far from it.* Does it mean we shouldn't step back and look at the bigger picture of *why* we have so much confusion, anger, resentment, miscommunication, disrespect, and

---

42   I adapted this from Lauren Nelson's essay "So You're Tired of Hearing about 'Rape Culture'?" here: rantagainsttherandom. wordpress.com/2013/03/19/so-youre-tired-of-hearing-about-rape-culture/

physical abuse? No. Women do get sexually assaulted, more often than many would like to admit and more than we would like to hear about. According to the documentary *The Hunting Grounds* about sexual assault on college campuses, a compilation of several research studies found that only 4 to 8 percent of rape accusations are false—which means that *at least* 92 percent of them are true.

It is absolutely unacceptable to knowingly falsely accuse someone of rape or sexual assault. But if you're one of the people who is quick to point to the cases where men were falsely accused, I ask you to consider *why* you are more likely to focus on those less common cases. Is it because it makes you feel safer? Is it because having empathy for a female victim is harder for you than feeling the injustice experienced by a male victim? The victim and the accused are both important to consider, but why elevate one consistently over the other if it doesn't match the facts and statistics? Is it because you believe what you've been taught by this rape culture, that women really do want the sexual encounter, or that they are responsible or should be blamed? Sometimes it is easier to blame someone than to sit deeply with a discomfort that challenges us to reconsider our beliefs.

The blaming and shaming of rape victims still prevails in our culture. Women often remain silent after a rape because they fear that they won't be believed, or that they are to blame, or because they're confused about whether their experience really was rape.[43] There is also a lot of misunderstanding around what constitutes consent versus

---

43   Nicole M. Heath et al., "Silent Survivors: Rape Myth Acceptance in Incarcerated Women's Narratives of Disclosure and Reporting of Rape," *Psychology of Women Quarterly* 35, no. 4 (2011): 596–610.

sexual coercion. Many women question whether it can still be considered rape if they wanted to engage in some of the sexual activity, or experienced physical sexual arousal during the act, or if the event happened with a partner or spouse. This is why affirmative consent initiatives have begun across the country, in an effort to make clear that these circumstances might indeed be considered nonconsensual, depending on the context.

There are also, as we have seen, substantial differences in the sexual realm between women and men, and these differences can have potentially dangerous implications. For example, in a dating situation, psychology researchers found that men were more likely to over-perceive a woman's sexual interest, particularly if she was considered physically attractive. Women, on the other hard, were more likely to under-perceive a man's sexual interest.[44] On a related note, when women are sexually objectified, they are viewed as less human than men and less competent overall.[45] And studies have shown that when men view images of sexually stereotyped women in video games, they develop a greater acceptance of sexual harassment.[46] The number of ways in which we are impacted by sex and

44   Carin Perilloux, Judith A. Easton, and David M. Buss, "The Misperception of Sexual Interest," *Psychological Science* 23, no. 2 (2012): 146–151.

45   Nathan A. Heflick and Jamie L. Goldenberg, "Objectifying Sarah Palin: Evidence that Objectification Causes Women to Be Perceived as Less Competent and Less Fully Human," *Journal of Experimental Social Psychology* 45, no. 3 (2012): 598–601.

46   Karen E. Dill, Brian P. Brown, and Michael A. Collins, "Effects of Exposure to Sex-Stereotyped Video Game Characters on Tolerance of Sexual Harassment," *Journal of Experimental Social Psychology* 44, no. 5 (2008): 1402–1408.

gender expectations and limitations is neverending, and unfortunately none of us are immune to it.

What is Sexy?

Who is allowed to be sexy? This may sound like an odd question, but I think that our social beliefs do not overtly allow all women, of all colors, shapes, sizes, and ages, to be deemed sexy. Some women don't even have the social right to present themselves in "sexy" ways without others responding with judgment or disgust. For example, at Halloween I read an article about sexy costumes that asked what age is too old for a woman to dress in a sexy way for Halloween. Clearly "older" women are not supposed to present as sexy.

We have a strange understanding of sex appeal in our society. For a woman, it's more tied to how she appears to others than it is to how sexual she actually feels. Imagine a young, thin woman wearing a tight dress and high heels and revealing her cleavage. She would generally be deemed sexy. However, this appearance has nothing to do with how sexual she feels, whether she wants or likes sexual activities, or how in tune she is with her body when she is involved in sexual activities. This means that for women, appearing sexy may have nothing to do with actually being sexual.

Since it has become "cool" for girls to like porn, strip clubs, or exposing their bodies, we've seen a shift to what author Ariel Levy calls "raunch culture."[47] She describes this as the glorifying of a "red-light-district culture,"

---

47 Ariel Levy, *Female Chauvinist Pigs: Women and the Rise of Raunch Culture* (London: Pocket, 2005).

and writes about how this exhibitionism has become one definition of women's sexual liberation or empowerment. This red-light-district culture includes strip clubs, flashing breasts at Mardi Gras, watching pornography, "Girls Gone Wild" videos, acting like a porn star in the bedroom, and sleeping with as many people as possible.

I'm not saying that these activities are bad in and of themselves—such acts may indeed feel liberating, empowering, and pleasurable for plenty of women. But I think we need to ask: Who is defining this behavior as sexy or empowering? Why are some of these "sexual role models" actually women who are being paid to have sex and fulfill male fantasies? For them, sex is work, their job, even for the sex workers who enjoy the sexual activity. We need to question whether and in what circumstances sexual exhibitionism and fantasy performance create sexual liberation and empowerment, and when they don't. I believe that dressing, behaving, and interacting to fit into a specific ideal of sexual availability to men carries the danger of being disempowering if women have not considered whether their motivations for doing so are centered in their own pleasure, innate worthiness, and well-being.

Another component of sexiness, which I'll go into in more detail in later chapters, involves body image. Body image is how we assess the appearance of our bodies, both positively and negatively. If you grew up in America, you're quite aware of many negative messages about women's bodies, particularly about weight and size, blemishes, graying hair, cellulite, and wrinkles. As girls and women, we learn that much of our worth is determined by others and is based on our appearance. From television shows to movies, magazine ads to video games, a young, thin, white ideal of beauty is everywhere. How we navigate these ideal images and negative messages has a large impact on our sexual expression and comfort with sex. For example, one research study found that watching prime-time television shows and soap operas had a negative impact on young women's concept of themselves as sexual women.[48]

A component of this that is even more specific to sexuality is how we feel about the appearance of our genitals. How we perceive our vulvas, and what we assume is "normal" in terms of smell, shape, size, color, etc., can impact how comfortable we are being naked with a partner, as well as whether we are comfortable receiving oral sex. Indeed, it seems that the prevalence of pornography in today's world means that young women are exposed to an "ideal" picture of the vulva that does not match the vast and beautiful variety of actual vulvas in the world. Labiaplasty, or surgically altering the lips of the vulva to look "neater" and smaller, has been on the rise.[49] This has nothing to do with pleasure, but is primarily about how it looks to others (and occasionally about physical discomfort). I don't know about you, but in general I don't think that labia are meant to look "pretty"—they're meant to protect our urethra and vaginal opening and to make us feel good! I discuss this a bit more in chapter 5.

---

48   Erin J. Strahan et al., "Victoria's Dirty Secret: How Sociocultural Norms Influence Adolescent Girls and Women," *Personality and Social Psychology Bulletin* 34, no. 2 (2007): 288–301.

49   David Veale et al., "Psychological Characteristics and Motivation of Women Seeking Labiaplasty," *Psychological Medicine* 44, no. 03 (2013): 555–566, doi:10.1017/s0033291713001025.

Not surprisingly, women who are interested in masturbating, who regularly see a gynecologist, who check out and examine their own genitals, and who use a vibrator—these women score higher on a measurement of their genital self-image.[50] The more comfortable you are taking care of yourself, in terms of both health and pleasure, the more you like your genitals. And the more you like your genitals, the more likely you are to take care of yourself in multiple ways. Which comes first? I don't know. But changing the equation on either side can break the negative cycle of disliking and disrespecting your genitals.

Acceptance of Sexual and Gender Orientation Differences

Although lesbian, gay, bisexual, transgender, and queer folks have been gaining status and respect in our country, there is still a stigma for many in the LGBTQ community, and especially for young people who realize they don't fit in with mainstream expectations. The shame and fear can have devastating results. Gay, lesbian, and bisexual teens are almost five times more likely than straight teens to attempt suicide.[51] This is a national crisis that needs to be taken seriously and addressed through compassionate education. Millennials and Generation Z folks have a greater acceptance of more fluid understandings of

50   Debby Herbenick et al., "The Female Genital Self Image Scale (FGSIS): Results from a Nationally Representative Probability Sample of Women in the United States," *The Journal of Sexual Medicine* 8, no. 1 (2011): 158–166.

51   Laura Kann et al., "Sexual Identity, Sex of Sexual Contacts, and Health-Related Behaviors among Students in Grades 9–12—United States and Selected Sites, 2015," *MMWR Surveillance Summaries* 65, no. 9 (2016): 1–202.

sexuality, gender, and love, which leads to greater toler-ance. But despite the greater acceptance by younger genera-tions, I believe that when any one group is oppressed in their sexual or gender expression, despite that expression being healthy and consensual and loving, it can bring down the sexual freedoms and fulfillment of an entire society.

Why do some people care what other people do in their bedrooms or their relationships? I think it boils down to our societal fears around the power of sexual expression, and a discomfort and shame around our bodies. When people don't fully accept themselves as the sexual beings they are, they don't behave well toward others who do. It's unfortunate and unjust when those people are in positions of power to decide policy, laws, or religious standards concerning sex education, marriage, and civil rights. Injustice around sex and gender for anyone is an injustice for all of us.

WHO TEACHES US MADNESS?

We receive negative messages about our sexual bodies from so many directions. This can include our parents or guardians, siblings, neighborhood friends, schoolteachers, religious leaders and texts, magazines, TV shows, the news, music lyrics and videos, movies, billboards, the internet, porn, and our personal sexual experiences with others. The messages we receive as women tend to be at polar extremes: One message demands that we be virgins, moral, and responsible; the other demands that we be porn-star insatiable. Add in the twentieth-century romantic notion that we're supposed to find our ultimate fulfillment through sex with a lifelong partner, and it's a lot of pressure!

Although I've listed many sources that may have taught you negative things about sex, I'm going to dive into three specific areas, so you are able to reflect more deeply on the sources of such messages and the impact they have had on you personally. This doesn't mean that you haven't also received positive messages, maybe from empowering media or knowledgeable family members. But the intent of this chapter is to shed a bright light on what you might have learned and still carry with you, lessons that block your ability to be more open in your sexuality.

Family of Origin

Do you remember the earliest references to sex or sexuality in your household? I've talked to some female clients who only ever heard sex referenced via the following warning: "Do not come home to this house pregnant." For an adolescent girl, the takeaway of a message like this is that she cannot trust her parents as resources for sexual information. Others grew up with parents who never mentioned anything about sex, so the subject was embarrassing because of its noticeable absence. On the other end of the spectrum, I've talked to some women who had mothers or fathers who were nurses, doctors, or health educators who made sure that their kids knew a lot about their anatomies and sex. Some of these kids grew up to be very comfortable with the topic. But others were embarrassed by how open their parents were; they saw that the rest of society wasn't so open.

Do you know what messages your parents or guardians were raised with concerning sex? Did they just pass on their own lack of education around the topic, or did they break the mold of what they were taught? This cycle matters. Your family loved you, and they raised and protected you in the best way they knew how. But you can't help but pick up values and beliefs that your family had, and if you aren't aware of them, you might unwittingly pass them on to the next generation. Mindfulness, however, can help you have a choice about that.

Religion

While there is a great variety of attitudes toward sexuality in religious beliefs, many organized religions emphasize the morality component of sexuality. Religious authorities expect that such dogmas will be internalized by believers, who ideally will only engage in approved sexual thoughts and activities. As a result, many positive aspects of sex, from intimacy and deep connection to exploration and pleasure, are only discussed in terms of a morally approved heterosexual marriage. These religious beliefs become so deeply ingrained that they control our behavior and emotions behind closed doors. Talk about a powerful impact!

Were you raised in a specific religion? If so, what did you learn about sex? What is your earliest memory of hearing about anything sexual in a religious context? Sometimes the sexual messages can be mixed or inconsistent. For example, my mother was raised Catholic, and when she was around eighteen years old and dating the man who would eventually become her husband and my father, she spoke to a priest in confession. She confessed that she had allowed a boy to inappropriately touch her. The priest responded: "But is he Catholic?" When my mother responded that he wasn't, she was given a harsher penance of five Our Fathers and five Hail Marys.[52]

Religion is also a part of our lives through which we can get a lot of strength, as well as a sense of community, purpose, and goals. This matters in our complicated and sometimes painful world, with all its suffering and uncertainty. You may be reading this and wondering how to hold on to your religious beliefs and values while also feeling open to accepting and exploring yourself as a sexual woman. In my dissertation research on HIV prevention programs, one of the educators I interviewed in New York City shared how she approached this topic with the many Christian women with whom she worked. She pointed out that if God hadn't intended sex to be so pleasurable, the clitoris so sensitive, and the deep connection we get with another through sexual intimacy so significant, he wouldn't have made us that way! I think the best personal approach to this is to consider what values and strengths you get from your religious beliefs and how they improve your life. Then consider what kind of shame or guilt you carry based on your religious beliefs, and reflect on whether carrying such heaviness helps you be a better person and more in service to your religion—or whether it gets in the way of you bringing the best of your unique gifts to the world. See where you can give yourself permission to forgive and love yourself as a sexual woman.

---

52 On a side note, my mother shared a particularly positive story about speaking to a priest during Pre-Cana, the Catholic premarital classes. My mother asked the priest what a married couple is to do if they do not want to have children right away, since the Church is against birth control. He responded: "You do what you have to do." She was incredibly grateful that she was given permission to take care of their sexual health needs without having guilt.

The Media

The media plays a particularly insidious role in what we learn about our bodies and our sexuality, because we're often not even aware that we're learning it. We often think that we don't notice advertisements, or that television or videos are just fun but not impactful. Research repeatedly shows that this is not the case.[53] Social norms, belief systems, gender roles etc., are all learned through how we see others portray those roles. Think about that fifteen-year-old girl from the beginning of this chapter as she learns about sexual expectations. No one directly teaches her the sexual norms of dating, but she learns what is expected of her from all around her. From the misogynistic song lyrics she listens to when she gets ready in the morning, to the cosmetic surgery billboards she passes on the way to school, to the thin models on her Instagram feed she scrolls through at lunch, to the romantic comedy she sees that evening with her friends, she is learning the expectations for behavior and appearance from everything around her. Unless we are taught how to be critical of the messages and values that are prevalent in mass media, we will passively absorb more than we realize. I address this exact skill-building in the Cultivate Media Literacy section of chapter 6.

I'd like you to reflect on what you remember about sexual imagery and how women's bodies were portrayed when you were growing up. For example, was there a billboard in your town showing a woman lying down in a bikini, an image used in an attempt to sell beer? Do you

---

53 Jane D. Brown and Susannah R. Stern, "Mass Media and Adolescent Female Sexuality," *Handbook of Women's Sexual and Reproductive Health* (2002): 93–112.

remember a sex scene from a movie with a woman who was easily pleased? Did you read in a book about how love conquers all, and that women should sacrifice their needs in the name of love? It's interesting and educational to reflect on what early media images may have shaped your beliefs about women and sexuality—and therefore about yourself.

The main negative impacts of all of this imagery are shame, embarrassment, guilt, disconnect, self-hatred, and fear. These emotions aren't sexy. Shame can bring us down in a lot of ways. Brené Brown writes, "If shame is the universal fear of being unworthy of love and belonging, and if all people have an irreducible and innate need to experience love and belonging, it's easy to see why shame is often referred to as 'the master emotion'."[54] Shame may drive women to avoid sex or intimate relationships, or may create low sexual desire, difficulty with arousal, or inability to orgasm. When you're feeling emotions like these, you're probably not comfortable stating your needs or indicating your preferences when having sex. You may believe that you need to perform to please your partner, but feel disembodied from your own arousal and pleasure. Whether on a small scale or a large scale, it's clear that we are taught many more negative ways to view being sexual than positive ones, and we can carry these messages within us for a long, long time.

EXPANDING YOUR COMFORT ZONE

What we learn about sex and gender growing up often centers on the "appropriate" ways to express ourselves and interact with others. For some, this emphasis on

---

54   Brown, *The Gifts of Imperfection*, 40.

"appropriateness" can create a rather small circle of comfort and acceptability. This book is about encouraging you to slowly expand your circle of comfort so that you can live a fuller, richer existence, a life that allows for greater self-expression, authenticity, connection, and fulfillment. As I stated in the Introduction, expanding your comfort zone requires a willingness to be vulnerable, which means being *un*comfortable. Why does it matter to push ourselves in these ways? Because these are the main areas about which people have regrets at the end of life. In an informal study, palliative care worker Bronnie Ware, who cared for people on their deathbeds for several years, heard five lifetime regrets. The people in her palliative care work wished they had worked less, stayed in touch with friends, allowed themselves to be happier, had the courage to authentically express emotions, and had the courage to live their lives in a way of their own choosing, not as prescribed by the expectations of others. [55] This is heavy stuff. I would venture to guess that dying with regrets is one of the biggest fears people have. Regarding regrets in the area of sexual intimacy, most of us have a lot of room for growth in our courage to express our emotions and to create a sexual life of our choosing, not one based on what we "should" do. Living a life like this is not easy, for it evokes discomfort and does require courage. But the easy path in life rarely results in fulfillment in the long run. Plus, the more we push outside our comfort zones, the more creativity and resiliency we build; this allows for a genuine love of our lives.

---

55 Bronnie Ware, *The Top Five Regrets of the Dying: A Life Transformed by the Dearly Departing.* (Bloomington, Ind.: Balboa Press, 2011).

Noticing discomfort, and then choosing to be curious about it instead of running from it, is quite counter to how we instinctively react. We naturally want to protect ourselves from this pain of discomfort, whether physical or emotional. Even seeing someone we care about in pain evokes visceral discomfort for us. I think this explains the "I'll kill him" response of so many men when a woman close to them shares a story about being sexually assaulted. Generally, what such a woman needs most is compassion, support, listening, and nurturing. But the immediate retribution response comes from a fix-it mode, which is a way of distancing oneself from pain. There are many other ways, too, that people self-protect from pain, such as blaming others, emotionally shutting off, or changing the topic and distracting their minds. Self-numbing, through alcohol, drugs, or food, is also a common choice.

There are a lot of reasons why we might feel discomfort with sexuality: the negative messages, the contradictory messages, the confusing messages, the messages of shame, the messages that we're in some way broken. These all have a strong influence on shaping our sexual experiences and even how much we like ourselves. You may have a narrow range of tolerance for feeling discomfort around some of these topics. But this is where mindfulness comes in. This is where you need to dig in to your courage to start cultivating mindfulness around sexual topics.

In the spring of 2016, I earned my black belt in Soo Bahk Do, a Korean martial art. As a sociologist, I appreciate learning about cultural and language differences. The word "courage" in Korean is "yong gi." One of my instructors taught that although it translates to "courage," it actually means something more like "brave energy." I like this. It helps me see that courage isn't a lack of fear; it's about accessing and cultivating my brave energy. When I had to break a board with a jump spin back kick as part of my black belt testing, I was filled with fear. What the hell was I thinking, as a forty-three-year-old woman, doing martial arts and trying to break a board three quarters of an inch thick with my bare heel? But I realized it was okay for my fear to coexist with a trust in myself—and that even if I messed up, I would still be okay. That was my brave energy.

A large part of my intention in this book is to expand your comfort zone and help you find this courage in yourself. Your comfort zone is the patterns of behavior you often unwittingly cling to because you believe they will keep you safe from stress or fear or pain. In the book *The Untethered Soul*, author Michael A. Singer explains: "You think, 'I am a woman. I am of a certain age and I believe in one philosophy versus another.' You literally define yourself based on what you believe. . . . But it is not who you are. It is just the thoughts you have pulled around yourself in an attempt to define yourself."[56]

Please know that I don't mean this in the vein of "You don't like anal sex? Push through that and get over it already!" Not at all. Singer explains how we create our own cages in life. Our comfort zone is cozy and designed to our liking and important for us to be able to have anxiety-free time—but even if it has comfortable blankets and plush pillows scattered about, it is still a cage. This is how most of us live our lives, and how most women are

---

56 Michael A. Singer, *The Untethered Soul: The Journey beyond Yourself* (Oakland, Calif.: New Harbinger Publications, 2007), 130.

taught to behave sexually. We end up locking ourselves into a limited range of sexual expression. But to change that, we'd have to venture into the unknown, and that scares us.

Paying attention to the sensations around your "heart center"—the center of your chest—can help you notice whether you are staying open to challenging your comfort zone or are closing down to new and uncomfortable experiences. The heart center is an area of your body with emotional neural pathways to your brain, and it's an area where you feel deep emotions, often through sensations of constriction or expansion. Singer writes, "When your heart starts to close, just say, 'No. I'm not going to close. I'm going to relax. I'm going to let this situation take place and be there with it.' Honor and respect the situation, and deal with it."[57] Although it might sound counterintuitive, it was "heart-opening" practices like this that helped me shift from "I don't love parts of me" (which I wrote about in the Introduction) to loving all of myself, even the messy, work-in-progress parts. It's an ongoing process of accepting all of myself in any given moment, despite what societal messages tell me I should or shouldn't love.

Singer's description above is what I mean by "staying present" with uncomfortable emotions. By staying present, you can actually learn to have a choice about whether to be open or closed to challenging situations. I want you to consider: Do you tend to stay open even when it feels scary, or do you shut down, in a restrictive retreat? A quick way to experience this difference is to imagine hugging a person or animal that you love. Or imagine that

---

57   Singer, *The Untethered Soul*, 46.

they have done something that you're really proud of. Can you feel the opening and warmth in your heart center? Now try to remember a time when you were so angry that you wanted to punch someone or act out physically in some way, or perhaps a time when you found out your partner was cheating on you. Can you feel the tightening in your chest? Did the first visualizations feel expansive, and did the second ones feel restrictive? Play with these visualizations and sensations for a little bit, as they'll help you throughout the rest of this book to recognize the difference between feeling open and feeling closed. Developing an awareness of these kinds of visceral sensations is helpful in identifying when you are pushing the boundaries of your comfort zone and therefore creating the potential for growth.

As you've done throughout this chapter, now consider what you learned about sex growing up, your current beliefs around it, and what fears or discomforts arise when you think about it. Do you feel your heart opening or closing? This is what I mean by pushing your comfort zone—questioning what you've been taught to believe and asking why you have the emotional responses that you do. Then you can consider how your comfort zone may actually be holding you back from happiness.

Although the 2005 movie *Prime* wasn't my favorite, there was a great line in it, spoken by Uma Thurman: "Get messy in life—at least you know you're living." This is what I'm talking about here. If you've been taught to be a good girl, follow the rules, stifle your dreams in the pursuit of pleasing others, and avoid judgments, then getting messy is probably outside your comfort zone. And this means a lot more than physical messiness. It involves entering new territory and taking risks mentally, emotionally, socially, and spiritually. While expanding your comfort zone may be uncomfortable, especially at first, this process is ultimately about leaving the madness behind and pursuing your version of happiness. This kind of pursuit of pleasure, when emanating from a pure drive for connection, love, appreciation, and joy, gives us a taste of the best aspects of being human. Such pleasure requires the brave energy it takes to be completely honest with ourselves. Mindfulness helps us drop into that level of raw honesty, and to do it at a pace that is right for each of us.

REFLECTION & WRITING

What topics in this chapter resonated most deeply with you? Why?

....

....

....

....

....

....

....

What did you learn about sex and sexuality as a child? Was it positive?

....

....

....

....

....

....

....

....

What do you remember about your experience of "losing your virginity"? How was that defined?

....

....

....

....

....

....

....

....

What do you wish someone had told you or taught you about your sexuality?

....
....
....
....
....
....
....
....

Is it common for you to have negative thoughts about your body or sexuality? What are those most common thoughts?

....
....
....
....
....
....
....
....

What are your biggest fears around sex?

....
....
....
....
....
....
....
....

What is your vision of a happy sex life? What does it feel like? What would a happy sex life provide for you that you don't have now?

....
....
....
....
....
....
....
....

★ ACTION ITEM ★

Choose one female relative and two female friends and discuss questions 1 through 4 above with them. Practice vulnerability by sharing your responses as well.

CHAPTER 2

THE POWER OF MINDFULNESS

S eventeen couples sat in the hotel conference room, filling the small space for my couples' intimacy evening in February. These were executives and leaders, and their intimate partners, all dressed in business suits or stylish dresses.

Nervous laughter and whispers had punctuated the couples' activities that we had already done; this ninety-minute workshop was not for the faint-hearted. The topic was "Emotional and Physical Intimacy," which requires being mindful, open, and vulnerable. But vulnerability, especially for men, is hard. I expected that with this group of high-powered men, it would be even harder, despite the happy hour cocktails. With a fluttering of anxiety in my chest, I was feeling a bit of my own vulnerability, hoping that the activities wouldn't be interpreted as too cheesy by this crowd.

"For our next activity, I'd like you to give brief hand massages to each other," I began. "Choose who will give and receive first. I ask that the giver stay very present with what it feels like to touch your partner's hand and to just *give* to them. For the receiver, I ask that you be aware of what it feels like to receive, with no expectations. I have scented hand lotion up here if you'd like some."

I heard a smattering of giggles again. No one asked for lotion. One couple quietly excused themselves, whispering that they had actually wanted to go to one of the other workshops. Their obvious discomfort had been adding to the anxious feelings in my chest, so I was happy with their choice. The remaining couples settled into the activity, with one partner giving a hand massage, and the other receiving.

Despite the movement between couples, there was a stillness in the room. I stood quietly in the front, my eyes averted so as not to intrude on this PG activity that still felt so intimate. And then something changed. I felt my shoulders drop a couple of inches. With a deep exhale, I relaxed into my body. I could feel an opening in my heart, a spreading warmth of love and appreciation, which I immediately attributed to a shift in energy in the room. The couples were dropping emotionally into this practice as their walls of protection fell away. One pair gently smiled at one another. Another couple was inhaling and exhaling in unison, a carryover from a previous activity. I could actually feel in my own body the appreciation and love in the room, and I was grateful to share in their love on this Valentine's Day.

"Now I'd like for the giver to ask specific and concrete questions about what your partner likes," I calmly instructed. "For example, instead of asking a general question, like 'Does this feel good?' ask instead, 'Do you like *this* pressure, or *that* pressure better? Does it feel better when I rub you in *this* area of your hand, or this *other* area?' The receiver can then give detailed responses about their preferences. There's no right or wrong, just clear, mindful communication."

I could overhear murmurs of requests and responses. "I would have never guessed you liked that," one man whispered. The receivers also seemed emboldened to make specific requests. "Actually, could you just focus on deep pressure in this area?" one woman asked. Through this simple, everyday activity, they were learning skills in how to be present and nonjudgmental with each other.

• • • • •

I believe mindfulness is the foundation for all personal growth, especially in the intimacy realm. Are you embarrassed about asking for what you like in bed? Mindfulness can help break that fear pattern. Are you distracted during sex by your bulging belly or your long to-do list? Mindfulness skills can keep you grounded in the moment and release such insecurities or mind chatter. Has your desire for sex severely diminished in your relationship? Cultivating mindfulness can help you attune yourself to your body's desire and arousal and communicate such nuanced needs to your partner. Integrating little daily practices of mindfulness can help you make these big changes. Like the couples in the story above, even small mindfulness exercises can create space for intimacy and deeper connection.

You may have misconceptions about what mindfulness is or is not, so in this chapter, I clarify the most common misunderstandings and offer a lot of information and informal practices for mindfulness that you can do in your own home and integrate into everyday life. While the concept of mindfulness is simple, the actual practice of it can be frustratingly difficult. But this doesn't mean you won't quickly start to notice positive changes in your life. Dive in—I think you're going to like this!

WHAT IS MINDFULNESS?

Mindfulness is both the simplest concept and the most difficult practice. Don't let this scare you away from it, though, because its power to transform your life is profound. It takes time to learn, but there are many small, simple practices that are immediately beneficial. Here's a formal definition of mindfulness: "The effort to attend, nonjudgmentally, to present-moment experience, and to sustain this attention over time, with the aim of cultivating stable, nonreactive, metacognitive awareness."[58] A shorter definition is that mindfulness is focused awareness in the present moment, without judgment.

However, I want to add a piece to this definition that is missing from some other approaches: compassion. A great example of mindfulness without compassion is a sniper—laser-focused in the moment, without judging their thoughts or activities. Mindfulness with compassion, on the other hand, includes caring about your suffering and the suffering of others. The combination of the two can positively change individual lives, and the world.

As a concept and philosophy, mindfulness has been

---

58   Eric Garland and Susan Gaylord, "Envisioning a Future Contemplative Science of Mindfulness: Fruitful Methods and New Content for the Next Wave of Research," *Complementary Health Practice Review* 14, no. 1 (2009): 3–9, doi:10.1177/1533210109333718

practiced for many thousands of years. Our under-standing of mindfulness is culled primarily from ancient Buddhist teachings, but at its core it is not about religion. The pure presence of mindfulness can be beneficial to anyone. At the core of the practice is recognizing that the past has already happened and the future hasn't happened yet, so all we have is right now. And now. And now. This moment. This fleeting moment is all that exists.

When you can focus your awareness to the present moment and observe what is happening to you and around you *without judgment*, you can access a depth of knowing that wasn't previously available. By "depth of knowing," I mean a greater awareness of your emotional and physical reactions to the world inside you and outside you, and how those reactions influence your beliefs and actions. The more you know yourself, the more empowered you are to make healthy decisions and satisfying choices. This is beneficial in all parts of your life.

Let me offer an example. Have you ever been unhappy on a Sunday evening or on the last day of a vacation? You're probably thinking about the next day when you have to return to work, instead of the situation and moment you're actually in. In the moment, you could be enjoying and appreciating your time off. But instead, you are missing the joy in the moment and dragging future worry into the now.

We all live with a lot of chaos in our brains. Often we don't even know it because we're on automatic pilot, moving through life just reacting and thinking and feeling and reacting some more. We have a voice that goes on and on in our heads, providing commentary about the world, judging whether it's good or bad to us. If you just thought to yourself, "What voice?", *that's* the voice I'm talking about.

Imagine that you're walking along a river in a beautiful wooded setting, enjoying the red and yellow leaves and the crisp fall air. You're appreciating the present moment. Suddenly you have a thought about a work email you received that morning, and you feel your chest tighten with anxiety because you're afraid that you might be in trouble with your boss. It's like you were standing on the river's shore, and suddenly you're being tossed about in the middle of the raging river. Your constant mind chatter and seemingly uncontrollable emotions are like that raging river, which keeps sweeping you away from the present moment. It's all you know—it's all your brain knows how to do unless you train it differently.

So what if you had the choice to stand on the edge of that river, with only your feet feeling the chaos of the water, and observe the river of thoughts and emotions as it passes? You could be fully aware of what is going on, but not get swept up in it. When you recognize that you are not your thoughts, and that your emotions and feelings are passing entities, this creates new possibility. You have space to observe, grow, make choices. Sometimes you can even experience amusement about what's happening in the river, even while you feel the chaos at your feet. You are *observing while feeling* it in your body. (If this sounds too difficult, don't worry! I'm just sharing the *ideal* of mindfulness; the *practice* of it is forgiving and kind.)

I present a version of mindfulness here that focuses on developing awareness and acceptance that is culturally relevant to the experience of twenty-first-century American society. It is a process of learning to observe the happenings within *you*, from your thoughts, inter-pretations, beliefs, and mental distractions to your urges, emotions, and bodily sensations. In the past, all of this stuff going on inside of you led to patterns of behavior, and these may be getting in the way of having a happy relationship or sex life. In this way, your past continues to dictate your future.

Jon Kabat-Zinn, a professor of medicine emeritus, who has done tremendous work in bringing mindfulness into mainstream American society and the medical field, writes: "The habit of ignoring our present moments in favor of others yet to come leads directly to a pervasive lack of awareness of the web of life in which we are embedded . . . . It severely limits our perspective on what it means to be a person and how we are connected to each other and to the world around us."[59] Mindfulness is a process of becoming an observer of yourself through embodied awareness, not just a passive actor in your life. And when you are more mindful, you can connect more deeply to others. Developing mindfulness is much like building a muscle that needs to be stretched and strengthened slowly over time to become stronger and more powerful.

I teach applied mindfulness as a three-step process of the three A's: Awareness, Acceptance, and Action. When you choose to focus in the present, you may be surprised by how much has been going on beneath your general awareness, and how many alternative choices are avail-able to you. These three steps together can be remark-ably empowering when you have an emotional trigger—a

---

59   Jon Kabat-Zinn, *Wherever You Go, There You Are: Mindfulness Meditation in Everyday Life* (New York: Hachette, 2014), 5.

behavioral pattern that you currently have no control over. Examples of triggers are when you feel rushed and your child won't put on her shoes, and you can't stop yourself from yelling at her; you're lonely at nighttime and eat that nighttime snack even when you're not hungry; or you shut down emotionally and verbally when your partner says they feel disappointed in you. Let's take a closer look at each of the three steps.

1) **Awareness.** Awareness means shining a bright light on what's happening in the moment, in terms of your thoughts/beliefs, emotions, and bodily senses/sensations. The observer part of you—the part you consciously engage with when you're practicing mindfulness—helps you see that you *experience* your thoughts, emotions, or sensations, but you are not *defined* by them. This is the difference between being *in* the river, versus *watching* the river while still experiencing it. This distinction may seem confusing in the beginning, but after a short time of practicing it, this will make more sense and start to provide a calmer way to view your life. Later in this chapter, I share the Triangle of Awareness, which provides a visual aid to walk through this awareness process in much greater detail.

2) **Acceptance.** When you shine a bright light on this moment, you might not like what you see, find, and feel. This is exactly why we don't like to be so aware of the present moment—it can feel at the least uncomfortable, and at the worst terrifying and deeply painful. But accepting whatever you find, while having compassion for yourself as a loving parent would for their child, is exactly the process. Whatever you're experiencing can't be any

other way than the way it is in this moment, and resisting *what is* only causes more resistance and pain, not growth. It is not unusual for people to struggle with the acceptance part of mindfulness. You might believe that accepting these negative things about yourself and your life means you are condoning them or surrendering to them. Or that shining a light on them and accepting them means they will grow. This belief totally makes sense. However, our patterned responses actually work in the opposite way. Avoiding conscious reflection on them gives them power to grow, and reflecting on them is the first step in breaking their hold on you. And this is a vital step in learning to love *all* parts of you—even the parts that cause you pain.

It may also be difficult to accept those thoughts, emotions, or bodily sensations because you have been numbing them or running from them for many years. You have been distancing yourself from them for a long time because they are unpleasant. It can actually be physically painful to accept your flaws, imperfections, messiness, or "ugliness" as a human. (Note: We all have flaws and imperfections.) However, as Cheri Huber, a Buddhist teacher, writes, "Rejection does not lead to compassion. Compassion leads to compassion. Rejection leads to rejection. If you see something you don't like about the way you are and you beat yourself up for it, pretty soon you will have trained yourself to stop looking."[60] Rejecting any part of you means that you are not allowing the opportunity to accept all of who you are, which is an essential step to knowing you are worthy of self-growth and love.

---

60   Cheri Huber, *That Which You Are Seeking Is Causing You to Seek* (Mountain View, Calif: A Center for the Practice of Zen Buddhist Meditation, 1990), 10–11.

Tara Brach, PhD, author of *Radical Acceptance*, takes the concept of acceptance to an even deeper level. "Clearly recognizing what is happening inside us, and regarding what we see with an open, kind and loving heart, is what I call Radical Acceptance. If we are holding back from any part of our experience, if our heart shuts out any part of who we are and what we feel, we are fueling the fears and feelings of separation that sustain the trance of unworthiness. Radical Acceptance directly dismantles the very foundations of this trance."[61] Even if you do not like what you see, even if you find parts of yourself that frighten or disgust you, embracing all of you is necessary on the path of healing any past hurts. But this is not a mindset of complacency. It is a mindset of accepting what is showing up for you and making a new choice that is in harmony with your values and who you want to be as a healthy, fully expressed, and (in the context of this book) sexual woman.

3) **Action.** By action, I mean doing something different from what you would usually do in a triggered moment. The human brain, like that of all animals, strives to be efficient. This is why we can't help but have many automatic patterns. However, when we create some space to be aware of and accept the triggers for those automatic patterns, we give ourselves the opportunity to choose how to respond, instead of just reacting. This takes effort to slowly rewire the brain.

It may be shocking to even consider that you have the

---

61   Tara Brach, *Radical Acceptance: Embracing your Life with the Heart of a Buddha* (New York: Bantam Dell, 2003), 26.

choice to do something differently. I consider this the epitome of empowerment—realizing you have a choice in moments when you didn't even know you had a choice. Sometimes the choice you make in this third step of mindfulness is actually not to act, but to stay quiet in reflection. Pema Chödrön, my favorite author on mindfulness and compassion, writes, "Through refraining, we see that there's something between the arising of the craving—or the aggression or the loneliness or whatever it might be—and whatever action we take as a result. There's something there in us that we don't want to experience, and we never do experience, because we're so quick to act."[62] The first two steps of this mindfulness process show that you are not your thoughts, emotions, or sensations. They are part of you, but they do not define you, and you can accept that they are there whether you like them or not. The third step teaches that when you are able to take a step back and observe, you see you have some time and space to do something differently.

In the long run, I guarantee that mindfulness has the potential to make you happier and calmer. In the short run, though, when you're facing your life in new ways, it can feel intimidating and deeply unsettling. The gift of this discomfort, though, when you learn to stay present with it, is that you can then know how to live a life of intention and choice. This is very different from reactivity, which runs rampant in relationships and intimate interactions. This kind of personal growth is beneficial to all areas of your life. But since intimacy and sex are so taboo,

---

62   Pema Chödrön, *Comfortable with Uncertainty: 108 Teachings on Cultivating Fearlessness and Compassion* (Boulder, Colo.: Shambhala, 2002), 34.

it can sometimes take a bit more time and perseverance to get to the heart of transformation around these topics. This is why the Reflection & Writing sections at the end of each chapter, to assist in your growth in the sexual realm, are so important.

There is a delicate balance between acknowledging and accepting your negative feelings and thoughts, and being consumed by them. Ideally, the "acceptance without judgment" component means that you're fully feeling the discomfort but not getting stuck wallowing in it. I believe that wallowing sometimes gives us a sense of satisfaction because we are indulging in feeling unhappy. The real satisfaction you're looking for here, though, is in making that shift from "This feels bad, my life sucks, and I don't have any control over this" to "This feels bad, and I'm able to accept that this is part of what it is for me to be human. I can now act and make a different choice than I usually would." The integration of compassion (empathy in action) in the latter means these concepts are worlds apart.

Mindfulness helps you see your patterns and decide whether they are serving you. Your patterns and triggers are there for a reason; you learned at some point in the past to protect yourself from some unbearable feeling, sensation, or belief. But the question to consider now is whether that pattern is serving the best version of you, making you happy in the long run, and allowing you to connect authentically with others.

WHAT IS MINDFULNESS NOT?

It's not unusual to hear someone who has tried meditation or mindfulness practices say "I can't do it" or "I'm terrible at this." I think they say those things because they have a misconception about these practices. First of all, mindfulness is not the same as meditation, although practicing them together is helpful and powerful. As already stated, mindfulness is focused, nonjudgmental awareness in the moment. You can practice mindfulness at all times and in all interactions. Meditation is also focused awareness, but generally it is practiced in a formal way, such as the traditional seated meditation, or in a very slow, repetitive walking meditation.

I believe that a combination of informal practices in everyday life and formal practices in your free time is the best approach to cultivate mindfulness. However, the cultural context of American society does not easily facilitate such formal practices, so although I strongly suggest them, this book is focused primarily on more informal daily practices related to sex, bodies, intimacy, and relationships. Later in this chapter, I will walk you through several daily practices in mindfulness that are easily integrated into your busy schedule.

Another common misconception is that mindfulness (and meditation) is about "clearing your mind." This belief unfortunately leads many people to believe that mindfulness is impossible for them, because they experience their thoughts as constant, scattered, and out of control. Mindfulness is not about clearing your mind, but about choosing to focus your attention, noticing when you're distracted, and then choosing to bring your attention back over and over again. You may only stay focused for three seconds at a time, and that's fine, as long as you eventually notice your distraction, don't attach negative value to being distracted, and choose to refocus. That's it. So, if you think about it this way, the more distracted you are and the more you have to refocus, the more you're working on mindfulness!

You may have heard about meditation experiences where an individual has hallucinogenic peak experiences, feeling transported to another time and place or suddenly grasping the meaning of the universe. That's not what this is about! This is about seeking insight into the everyday happenings of your own mind so that you may gain the ability to create new versions of your everyday happenings. The mindfulness discussed in this book is about how to observe your state of mind, with its accompanying emotions, feelings, and beliefs, and recognize that you can learn to shift it over time if it's not working for you. Through mindfulness you can learn to observe and study your own mind.

One last common misconception about mindfulness is that it should be relaxing or lead to immediate happiness. This is most certainly not the case. As you'll learn in this book, practicing mindfulness is often difficult and uncomfortable. Being present and aware in new ways is a challenging experience for many. It can feel disconcerting to seemingly be doing nothing while being alone with your own mind and body. This may be the first time you're choosing to focus on certain thoughts, emotions, or sensations that you've been avoiding since childhood. This is hard. It can hurt and feel very scary. But knowing that you're choosing to do this for your long-term well-being will hopefully motivate you to face those fears. Cultivating mindfulness does not make your problems go away. It doesn't mean you never have new concerns. What changes is your relationship to your problems and your ability to trust in your resiliency to move through them.

This may sound like a small change, but it is huge in its potential for your happiness in life and fulfillment in relationships.

WHY MINDFULNESS IS SO HARD

Mindfulness can be particularly hard in today's world because we live in such a fast-paced society and are pulled in so many directions. We often live to work instead of work to live. We live in pursuit of some abstract happiness that we are told comes from material possessions or acquiring a specific status. But this "hedonic treadmill" keeps us always wanting more and never really moving forward in terms of sustainable happiness.

It's also hard because we are taught to distance ourselves from uncomfortable feelings. As discussed in chapter 1, there can be *a lot* of uncomfortable beliefs and feelings when it comes to sexual expression. That means we're often distracting, numbing, or distancing ourselves from being present with our sexuality, particularly if something isn't going smoothly in our sex lives.

What do we tend to do instead of being mindful? We worry, obsess, blame, react, or suffer. We feel shame and fear and ultimately are disconnected from acceptance of our true selves. This means we can't truly be present with someone else intimately, because we have our walls of protection up. And these walls do their job well, because they really do protect us and block us. But protections keep others out. This is the opposite of the vulnerability and presence needed to experience deep intimacy with others. I define the ideal of "deep intimacy" as connecting with another while cultivating mindfulness, compassion (for self and others), vulnerability, and authenticity. I think that one of the most extraordinary things we can share with another human is choosing to be vulnerable and raw, in all of our beauty and messiness as humans, and create a safe space for them to do the same.

As mentioned previously, I use the word "trigger" to refer to those moments when you feel like you have no control. Triggers show up in lots of places, and I believe that most of them are there for one of two reasons: 1) You learned a certain behavior by watching it repeatedly in a parent or someone close to you growing up, and it's the only reaction that makes sense to your brain in the moment, or 2) you learned that behavior as a way to protect yourself from a combination of really uncomfortable thoughts, emotions, and/or bodily sensations. As children, we have a very small toolbox from which to choose how to handle life's difficulties. If you're facing hurt, fear, neglect, or shame, the reaction you construct to make that feeling go away in that moment serves to protect you from discomfort. It also means that by the time you're an adult, whenever a person or situation evokes similar thoughts, emotions, or sensations, you will be triggered into your automatic pattern. Since our brains strive for efficiency, this pattern has become a particularly efficient path in your brain. When you practice mindfulness, you can access the core of both of these reasons for triggers, although I mention the latter with more frequency in this book.

The habits you formed at a young age have had a lot of time to become efficient. For example, did you learn that masturbation was not allowed in your household, and that it was shameful? Well, that belief has had many years to become an efficient neural pathway in your brain.

The good news is, it isn't cemented in your brain. We have brain plasticity—the ability to rewire our brains—until the day we die. Key to this, though, is making a conscious choice to do something differently, so you can start to create new neural pathways.

HOW MINDFULNESS WORKS

Here is a simplified version of how the benefits of mindfulness affect our brain. Mindfulness practices help develop new neural pathways in a part of our brain called the prefrontal cortex. This higher-consciousness part of the brain is sometimes referred to as the captain or CEO of the brain, since it's the seat of rational decision-making. Through intentional focus, this area allows us to gain some control over our lower-consciousness brain. Neural pathways connect the parts of our brain to each other, and also connect the brain to other parts of our body. Our triggers—which are just quick and efficient neural pathways within the body—stem from the natural stress response of fight, flight, or freeze and are strengthened over time with repeated use. But when we focus on something—which activates our prefrontal cortex—it can either further ingrain the existing pathways *or* allow us to start creating new pathways.

Mindfulness practices, which help create stronger neural pathways from the prefrontal cortex to the rest of the brain, increase our ability to notice what the mind is doing—in other words, to notice which neural pathways are firing and when we've been triggered in a stress response. When we increase our ability to observe the activity of our mind, it creates new neural pathways that are more of our choosing, based on focused attention, and allows the reactive, out-of-control trigger pathways to wither over time. When you step back and observe how your thoughts work, you start to have choices about how you respond to what pops up. This kind of control is a key element of emotional intelligence, and it can be incredibly helpful in cultivating healthy relationships. Through mindfulness practice, we can train the different parts of our brain to work together in a way that improves our emotional well-being.

I have really enjoyed Daniel Siegel's work on mindfulness and brain science and what he calls "mindsight." Mindsight refers to integration between the brain and body, a unity that allows for balance with ourselves and harmony with others. Siegel argues that practicing mindfulness leads to the development of nine traits or skills: "1) bodily regulation, 2) attuned communication, 3) emotional balance, 4) response flexibility, 5) fear modulation, 6) empathy, 7) insight, 8) moral awareness, and 9) intuition."[63] When we talk about being "emotionally mature" in relationships, this summarizes much of what we're referring to. These skills are all about being aware of what's going on for you with a calm awareness and acceptance, and also being aware of what's going on with others, with that same calm awareness. I think most of these skills are necessary for a sustainable, healthy relationship.

The brain stem, limbic area, and prefrontal cortex are the three primary areas of the brain relevant to a basic understanding of how mindfulness changes us. Daniel

---

63   Daniel J. Siegel, *Mindsight: The New Science of Personal Transformation* (New York: Bantam Books, 2011), 26.

Siegel simplifies it by literally putting the power to understand mindsight in the palm of our hand. In his research articles, books, and lectures, he instructs his audiences to hold a hand up, bend their thumb onto their palm, and close their four fingers over the thumb. (I encourage you to do this right now, and face your palm away from you, so that this represents the direction of your brain.) Your palm represents your brain stem, which regulates basic bodily functions and is often referred to as the reptilian brain. Your thumb (imagine, for greater accuracy, that you have a second thumb mirroring the first on the other side of your hand) represents the limbic system, best known for generating our fight, flight, or freeze response system. Your bent fingers represent your frontal lobe and, specifically, from your last knuckle down to your fingernails, they represent your prefrontal cortex.

Mindfulness practices create stronger neural pathways from the prefrontal cortex to the limbic system and brain stem, and between the left and right brain hemispheres. This is how mindfulness actually integrates and connects your brain in an intentional way. This is also how mindfulness helps you develop greater bodily awareness, regulation of your emotions, and choices in how to respond. This can have a profound impact. As Siegel writes, "Mindfulness appears to change how we see ourselves in the world. Indeed, our experience of the self changes with mindfulness."[64] The whole brain starts working together better. If you would like to learn more details, I highly recommend Daniel Siegel's work.

---

64   Daniel J. Siegel, "Mindful Awareness, Mindsight, and Neural Integration," *The Humanistic Psychologist* 37, no. 2 (2009): 146.

RESEARCH ON HEALTH AND SEX BENEFITS

While this book is about mindfulness as it relates to healthy and happy intimacy, I want to mention the researched health benefits of practicing mindfulness to provide a larger context. The greater our mental and physical health, the easier it is to put energy into our relationships and sexual expression. Also, many of these benefits are related to how we feel about ourselves and our interactions with others.

Research on mindfulness has exploded in recent years, and the benefits of mindfulness practices are well documented, although they are still being tested at the most rigorous levels of scientific study. Current research suggests that mindfulness practices can help overcome addictive behaviors and eating disorders, improve physical health (e.g., immune system, chronic pain),[65] and assist with mental/emotional health (e.g., stress, depression relapse, anxiety, ADHD, suicidal behavior). There are also positive correlations between mindfulness and many factors connected to overall well-being, such as life satisfaction, self-esteem, empathy, optimism, conscientiousness, and greater resilience to negative experiences.[66]

A study looking at couples who participated in a series

---

65   For an intense review of the latest research on mindfulness and physical health, check out this article: Linda E. Carlson, "Mindfulness-Based Interventions for Physical Conditions: A Narrative Review Evaluating Levels of Evidence," *ISRN Psychiatry* (November 2012): 1–21.

66   Read about many of the psychological benefits of mindfulness in this journal article: Shian-Ling Keng, Moria Smoski, and Clive Robins, "Effects of Mindfulness on Psychological Health: A Review of Empirical Studies," *Clinical Psychology Review* 31, no. 6 (2011): 1041–1056.

of mindfulness training classes found improvements in their level of closeness and abilities to relate to and accept each other. They reported that they felt they could better cope with stressors in the relationship. The researchers even found a direct positive link between higher levels of mindfulness practice and levels of relationship satisfaction overall.[67]

With such a long list of potential physical, emotional, and social benefits, mindfulness starts to sound like a panacea, doesn't it? While nothing is a cure-all, I do think cultivating mindfulness as an ongoing practice has the potential for substantial life improvements. (And as a side note, I personally believe that if compassionate mindfulness was cultivated from a young age, all around the world, we wouldn't have the wars, oppression, and divides that we do.) In the sexual realm, mindfulness is certainly not a magic pill or a quick fix, but when individuals and couples are willing to do the hard work of cultivating awareness and acceptance, they will likely reap the rewards.

Dr. Lori Brotto, a professor and researcher out of British Columbia, Canada, is the original and leading researcher on mindfulness as applied to women's sexual well-being. Through many research studies, she and her research teams have found that the use of ongoing mindfulness techniques improves multiple aspects of women's sexual experiences. Women experienced increased sexual desire and sexual arousal and reduced vulva pain and emotional distress from sex-related issues or past sexual trauma. She also found an increase in sexual satisfaction

---

67   James W. Carson et al., "Mindfulness-Based Relationship Enhancement," *Behavior Therapy* 35, no. 3 (2004): 471–494.

overall. These benefits seem to be related to two specific aspects of mindfulness training: greater awareness of subtle bodily sensations related to desire and arousal, and greater physical, mental, and emotional acceptance of whatever sex-related concerns the participant had. Dr. Brotto's medical- and psychological-based research has impacted the use of mindfulness in sex therapy practices around the world.[68]

Authors and psychology researchers Barry McCarthy and Lana Wald apply mindfulness to their concept of "Good Enough Sex" for couples. They write, "In the context of sex, the essence of mindfulness refers to the cognitive, behavioral and emotional awareness and acceptance of here and now sexual sensations and feelings."[69] This approach helps couples shift from the mainstream focus on sexual performance (where orgasm is often the only sexual goal) to a focus on sexual desire, awareness, and satisfaction in a sexual sharing process. Enjoying the journey of connecting deeply in the moment during sexual encounters is one of the huge gifts of mindfulness.

Sexual problems in a relationship can take a large toll on a couple's overall well-being, communication, and health, because they can undermine trust and connection. However, this doesn't have to be the case if the couple is open to creative and mindful solutions to address their concerns. One research study found a correlation between practicing mindfulness and being more open to seeking

---

68   Lori A. Brotto, *Better Sex through Mindfulness: How Women Can Cultivate Desire* (Vancouver: Greystone Books, 2018).

69   McCarthy and Wald, "Mindfulness and Good Enough Sex," 39–47.

novelty in sexual situations.[70] I think this is because practicing mindfulness helps us accept *what is* without judgment. This means we can address sexual concerns with a more open mind, instead of being fearful, blaming ourselves, or carrying resentment toward our partner.

What I glean from these studies and from my client work is that applying mindfulness creates more awareness and acceptance of sexual experiences, whether you would have labeled them as good, bad, or neutral. Mindfulness allows you to know more about what your body is doing and feeling at any given time. Such attuned awareness allows you to notice what feels good and stay present with that. And when something doesn't feel so good, you can shift your perception and take action if necessary, instead of ignoring or resenting those sensations. Whether you are distracted, worried about how your body looks, not feeling much desire, experiencing shame for being sexual, or carrying concerns about not being good enough, you have the opportunity to break from that stuck place and try something different.

If you recall the gender roles and sexual expectations outlined in chapter 1, you can probably imagine how this kind of attuned self-acceptance can reduce the unrealistic pressures around masculinity and femininity placed on both women and men. Mindfulness is also quite beneficial in the sexual realm because it can help you disengage from the pressure and expectation of specific goals (like orgasm) and open your mind and body to profound connection, play, and communication.

---

70   Asimina Lazaridou and Christina Kalogianni, "Mindfulness and Sexuality," *Sexual and Relationship Therapy* 28, nos. 1–2 (2013): 29–38.

THE TRIANGLE OF AWARENESS

One image I repeatedly use with clients to provide a more concrete anchor for practice is that of a triangle, as seen on page 80. This is the Triangle of Awareness that I have adapted from the mindfulness-based stress reduction course I took through the Center for Mindfulness at the University of California, San Diego.[71] In any moment, we may feel triggered and not in control of our thoughts or feelings. This indicates that an automatic pattern was invoked. This is quite normal. It's also normal to feel clueless as to how to stop these patterns. We can't just think our way through this; we also need to feel our way through it. This is where the Triangle comes in. Instead of feeling overwhelmed and out of control, like a boulder being pushed over the edge of a cliff, you can learn over time how to put some space and time between an emotional trigger and your reaction. Ultimately, over time, you can learn to have choice in the moment. As I've said before, I believe this is the epitome of empowerment—recognizing that you have a choice where you didn't before. With the Triangle, you are learning how to *respond* instead of *react*.

Any automatic pattern that you'd like to change has three distinct components. These happen quite fast, in no particular order, and they feed off of each other. They are:

_____

71   Eight-week mindfulness-based stress reduction classes are available throughout the country, and I highly recommend them. To learn more about the UCSD Center for Mindfulness, visit health.ucsd.edu/specialties/mindfulness The course content originated from Jon Kabat-Zinn's work at UMass Medical School Center for Mindfulness.

▸ Thoughts (your interpretation of what is going on and what it means to you)

▸ Emotions (such as embarrassment, fear, shame, or hurt)

▸ Bodily sensations (such as tightness, nausea, warmth, or butterflies in a specific location inside you)

As you'll see, by breaking down a reactive pattern into awareness about what's actually happening in the moment, and by choosing to focus your attention on your direct experiences (instead of running, numbing, shutting down, lashing out, or distracting), you can regain your power in that moment.

Let's dig into each component of the Triangle in more detail. Just considering that all of this is currently going on beneath your awareness level may be enough to shock your eyes wide open. There is no correct way to move through the Triangle, and no correct corner to start with. Just start with whatever stands out the most to you in any moment you're feeling triggered or out of control.

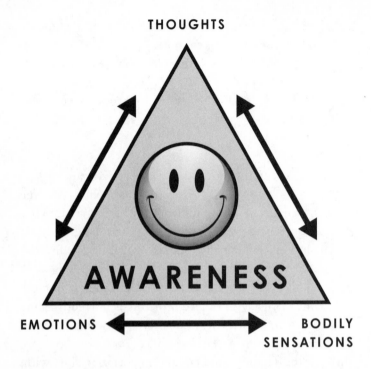

THOUGHTS

AWARENESS

EMOTIONS   BODILY
                           SENSATIONS

1) **Thoughts.** There are many components to your thoughts, including random observations about your day (e.g., I'm hungry, I should get a haircut, my friend is so funny), values and beliefs (e.g., sex outside of marriage is wrong; if I don't wear makeup to the gym, people won't find me attractive), and interpretations (e.g., he said my shoes look expensive . . . that must mean he thinks I'm superficial and spend too much money on clothing). Not all of this is on a fully conscious level. The cultural and family values that you learned at a young age will create a lens for interpretation and inform even random observations. For example, if you grew up hearing your mother compliment you only if she thought you were thin enough,

you may be much more likely to notice the size and shape of random women walking past and even mentally judge their worthiness by their weight. The most important point to glean from this part of the Triangle is that *you are not your thoughts*. I'm going to say that again—*You Are Not Your Thoughts*. Your thoughts happen to you, but they do not define you, even though it may feel that way. Think back to that "observer" self I referenced before, who is standing on the edge of the shore observing the raging river.

2) **Emotions.** Emotions are not well understood, even in the academic literature. We all have our own under-standing of emotions, and I think that's the best place to start. In general, emotions are feelings and states of being that we distinguish from reasoning or logical thinking. However, when I ask, "What are you feeling right now?" the majority of my clients respond with something along the lines of "I feel that he is being unfair." Or "I feel that I'm not valuable enough." These are actually thoughts and interpretations, at the top of the Triangle. But these statements are indicative of underlying emotions, such as sadness, fear, or anger. I actually hand out a long list of emotions to clients, broken into what we consider posi-tive and negative, to assist in identifying their emotions. This has proven quite fruitful in getting to the heart of a discussion. Some examples of common negative emotions that underlie patterns and triggers are sadness, hurt, disap-pointment, shame, worry, embarrassment, fear, and anger.

I want to take a moment to comment on anger as an emotion. I think anger has gotten a bad rap in some holistic and New Age circles, which is a shame. Anger is a wonderfully important emotion, and quite necessary in situations where your physical well-being or that of a loved one is threatened. We go astray with anger when we use it as a secondary emotion to mask deeper (and more uncomfortable) primary emotions. In such cases, mindfulness can help dig beyond the mask of anger to the other primary emotions that are fueling it.

For example, many men are taught that feeling and expressing emotions such as sadness or fear is weak and unacceptable. Can you imagine if little boys were all taught to own and articulate their emotions? "I'm feeling scared right now, and it's not okay that you're saying those hurtful things to me," or "This embarrassment is very uncomfortable—I feel like I want to throw up. But talking about it to you makes me feel a little better and know that I'm okay." It would be amazing. Although current cultural norms around appropriate gender roles don't encourage this, one by one, we can start modeling this for boys and young men.

Instead, in our society, little boys are teased, ridiculed, or humiliated out of the majority of their heavier emotions. However, anger and the emotions grouped with it, such as irritation, frustration, or annoyance, are socially acceptable for most men. As such, many men express anger in lieu of other underlying emotions. Anger feels powerful and like we're "doing" something with otherwise uncomfortable emotions. It makes sense that it's a go-to emotion programmed into many folks, including women.

Once, when I was working with a middle-aged couple, the man expressed his irritation that his girlfriend talked to her friends on a girls' night out about some of their intimacy struggles. I asked him to tell me what he was feeling, and he shared that constellation of anger-related emotions. When I asked what other emotions were present for him, he said none. Then I handed him the list of negative emotions with sixty-four nuanced emotions to choose from. He chose those same original emotions, but then also quietly articulated embarrassment, fear, and disappointment. A few tears rolled down his cheeks, something I did not expect from a man who had been in the military for over twenty years. I think he was surprised as well. He suddenly had insight into himself and the emotions at the core of his anger with his girlfriend. So anger should not be dismissed, but when it is surfacing as a secondary emotion, digging beneath that emotional layer can reveal the core concern.

3) Bodily Sensations. This is usually the hardest part of the Triangle for most people to understand, because when they are swept up in a moment, they don't notice what their body is doing or feeling. I think this is also the most powerful part of the Triangle for many people, because it is a new way of relating to themselves. Common bodily sensations include:

- Feeling like you've been punched in your gut
- Nausea in your belly
- A sinking feeling in your stomach
- Butterflies in your solar plexus
- Heaviness or a prickly feeling in your heart area
- Faster heartbeat
- Constriction in your throat
- Flushing in your face or ears
- A light-headed or fuzzy-headed feeling

▸ Warmth all over
▸ Tensed muscles

These are often quite uncomfortable sensations, and since they feel bad, we tend to quickly armor ourselves by lashing out, shutting down, or running away. Then, over time, we learn to fear even the potential of such bodily sensations and avoid situations that we think could cause them. For example, this is what procrastination is— avoiding something that we think will feel bad or will be uncomfortable in some way.

However, we can befriend these uncomfortable bodily sensations. Indeed, I believe befriending them is vitally important to personal growth. The more we know these sensations, the less abstract and scary they are. I've encouraged clients to go so far as to name their most unwelcome sensations with a human name. One female client felt exhausted a lot at work and also shared that she avoided confrontations. When we used the Triangle, we discovered that she avoided confrontation because she wanted to be nice and to be liked. She was, however, a manager at a high-stakes investment firm and needed to have difficult conversations to do her job well. The bodily sensation she was avoiding was primarily located in her chest and just below it, in her solar plexus. She described it as a murky orange cloud of heaviness that she named Nigel. This level of detail helped her own this discomfort. Moving forward, she was able to notice when it arose or when she was afraid it would arise, acknowledge it and compassionately allow it to exist, and then choose to breathe through it. Then she had the courage to face the confrontation she was avoiding. She also realized that resisting this process, instead of embracing it, had been leaving her exhausted. With this new self-knowledge, she was less avoidant of difficult conversations at work, and also less stressed with her responsibilities as a supervisor.

Here are some questions to guide you through becoming more intimate and accepting of these tough sensations. These abstract questions can actually create a concrete and almost tangible knowledge of your discomfort.

- ▸ Where do you feel the discomfort?
- ▸ What shape is it?
- ▸ What is the texture of that shape?
- ▸ How big is it?
- ▸ If it had a color, what color would it be?
- ▸ When do you first remember having this kind of feeling in your past?

Although these questions may sound crazy to you, I'm amazed how many people can answer them about their most scary reactions without hesitation. (Granted, I only choose to use this process with clients who I think will be open to visualizing in this way.) I think the most amazing part of the process is that the client always feels better after identifying the characteristics of these sensations, even when they are initially reluctant to do so. Then they are not frozen in avoidance and can choose a new path.

As another client example, I had been working with a heterosexual married couple in their early forties for a couple of years. They hadn't had sex in many years and didn't talk about it. He'd had an affair, and she'd discovered it shortly before they saw me. They were best friends, enjoyed sailing to exotic locations together, and had adopted three children. They loved and respected each other and didn't want a divorce, but didn't know how to rebuild trust, and certainly didn't know how to rebuild any physical intimacy. He was committed to moving forward, and at my suggestion, was willing to discuss his attractions to other women and be transparent about any contact he received from women in his past. This is a standard practice I recommend for couples trying to rebuild trust after infidelity. However, she needed to be able to be open and present in these conversations as well.

I worked alone with her many times, and we talked through her sexual triggers using the Triangle. She wanted to regain sexual intimacy with her partner, but didn't know what was blocking her. Her thoughts were that her husband wasn't attracted to her anymore and that her aging body didn't look as good as it had when they first met. She also thought that she shouldn't discuss sex with him or be vulnerable, and that she would lose self-respect if it seemed like she forgave his affair. Her emotions were fear, distrust, hurt, embarrassment, and humiliation. Her bodily sensations when discussing this included a constriction in her throat and nausea in her stomach area. This was a difficult process for her to sit through because it was scary, and it hurt emotionally and viscerally. But that's how she knew she was digging deep with courage— her brave energy—and carving a new path.

Just the process of getting this detailed about what sex with her husband meant to her, and choosing to face that discomfort instead of enacting her normal pattern of distracting and numbing, already started to give her space to be real with herself. Through acknowledging the embarrassment and humiliation, she realized that she needed to forgive herself first. She blamed herself for his affair, she realized, because she hadn't been interested in having sex. She was able to share these vulnerable emotions with him, do some journaling, and give herself permission to forgive herself. Doing this process gave her the strength and skills to have regular check-ins with her husband, so they could discuss his contact with other women. She started to develop trust and faith again, because her deepest discomforts weren't so scary anymore. Over time she was interested in trying some new, but safe, sensual activities with him.

INFORMAL PRACTICES

"When you begin the practice, the seed of mindfulness is quite small, but if you cultivate it every day, it becomes much bigger and stronger."[72] Vietnamese monk and peace activist Thich Nhat Hanh is so right. For most of us, mindfulness starts very small, because it is a new concept and worldview. However, with daily practice and small shifts, your awareness becomes stronger and applicable in more settings. Mindfulness is like a muscle, so attending to building its capacity every day, or nearly every day, is how you slowly shift to reclaim your power in your intimacy and relationships. And please note, when I write "reclaim your power," I mean the ability to enact positive change in your life, have choices where you didn't have them before, experience greater intimate connection, and feel proud of how you handle yourself.

Although the word mindfulness has "mind" in it, as

---

72   Thich Nhat Hanh, *You Are Here: Discovering the Magic of the Present Moment* (Boston, Mass.: Shambhala, 2012), 21.

you've already learned, the experience of mindfulness is much more of a full-body experience. I have had clients who believed that they had healed from their childhood emotional wounds by thinking their way through them. They applied their intellect without body awareness and believed they had moved beyond those patterns and reactions. These are often folks who are particularly uncomfortable with being vulnerable, and have convinced themselves they are healed, while unknowingly hiding behind their intellectual analysis. But breaking patterns and healing requires pulling back many layers of the onion, and bodily feedback and bodily wisdom are among those layers. So unfortunately, these folks stay stuck in their patterns.

I mention this leading into the section on practices because you cannot just read about mindfulness and expect to understand it, let alone gain the benefits of the practice. It must be experienced. The best frame of mind to cultivate when approaching these practices is one of curiosity. Be curious about what you can notice in the moment, what you can learn about yourself, and what can you observe in others. There is no competition, no finish line, nor any right or wrong. It is the journey of being in the moment. There is a freedom in being present in everyday moments. Just as with the hand massage activity in the story at the beginning of the chapter, bringing your intention and attention to any activity can break through your automatic pilot and allow for a deeper connection in any moment.

As you'll read in both the Informal and Formal Practices sections, focusing on your breath and your five senses are simple yet effective ways to develop mindfulness. Your breath and your awareness of your senses are always available to you, and therefore helpful when you want to pause whatever is happening in your mind and practice intentional concentration. Sometimes you will be instructed just to observe your breath, but other times the instruction is to take conscious deep breaths. Deep breathing, specifically through the nose, is a known strategy for reducing stress and giving pause to any pattern that might have been triggered. And since there is body movement involved with a deep breath, I often suggest it as a way of breaking your current train of thought and shifting focus to your body.

Stoplight Exercise

There are many ways to bring mindful awareness into how you move through the world. For example, you probably drive at some point during a typical day. You may feel frustrated when you're stopped at a red light, as it's impeding your efficient progress to reach your destination. But what if you used each red light as an opportunity to practice a few moments of awareness? What if you viewed that stoplight as a gift to your well-being? That shift in consciousness would be a powerful change in and of itself. Then, while you're sitting at the light, take three deep breaths—full in-breaths and out-breaths through your nose—as if that were the only moment that mattered. (Which, incidentally, it is.) Perhaps look around and find the brightest color that you can see around you. Observe the brightness of that color, without judgment of it or yourself. If you're distracted, notice that you're distracted, and choose to bring your focus back to observing your breath or that bright color. That's it. This is a small practice, but in this practice, you're choosing to harness intentional focus in the moment.

Doorway Breathing

What if every time you walked through a doorway, you took a deep breath and oriented yourself to the present moment? This would mean that many times a day you would be reducing stress and moving focus away from your ongoing thoughts and into your body—and consciously choosing to do so. If this practice sounds like it could be potentially beneficial, put a small sign above every doorway you typically walk through, with a reminder to breathe, smile, or slow down. This takes so little time out of your day and adds a lot in terms of self-nurturing and building presence of mind.

Mindful Eating

Since we eat several times daily, bringing a new focus to eating is a convenient way to start integrating mindful practices. Many of us have unfortunately been trained to eat on the run, whether in our cars, while working at the office, or after preparing dinner for our kids. Even eating while watching Netflix means you're not really paying attention to what's going into your mouth. There is so much joy available in the moment, especially when eating, if we pay attention to our five senses.

The next time you're eating, try this simple exercise. First, slow down when bringing the food to your mouth and eat at a slower pace than you normally do. Just as in the stoplight exercise, notice the colors in front of you. Then, pay attention to what you smell. When you bring the food to your mouth, what does it feel like against your lips? In your mouth? While chewing? What flavors are most prevalent? What do you hear while chewing? Your five senses are one of the best ways to anchor yourself in the present moment.

Are you appreciating your meal more now that you're paying focused attention to it? If you want to take this a step further in terms of appreciation, consider where this food came from, who grew it, raised it, cultivated it, transported it, put it in a grocery store or restaurant, and prepared it. And what land, water, and sun were needed to feed it. There is a lot involved in food production that we might take for granted. Regardless of the extent to which you take this activity, choosing to be mindful and appreciative is a very different way to move through a meal, and this awareness can carry over to other parts of your life. This kind of mindful eating is also healthier because it aids in digestion, reduces overeating, and encourages more conscious food choices.

Imagine if you brought this kind of appreciation and attention to your five senses to a sexual context? It's a powerful shift out of our heads and into sensuality and feelings of gratitude—which is what making love is all about. There is a specific practice I like to call "making love to an orange." It is the application of the five senses awareness mentioned above to eating an orange over a twenty-minute time period. This is great to do alone, or you can split the orange and share with your partner. If you slow down when eating an orange, you may notice that there are thousands of tiny juice pockets, each ready to explode with sweet juiciness. Let the juices run down your arms. Be messy and curious, like you're eating an orange for the first time. In some ways, you probably are. If you're doing this with a partner, lick the juice from each other's hands or face. The only goal is being present with your five senses and each other.

Mindfulness Bell App

One of my favorite daily reminders for mindfulness is a free mindfulness bell app on my phone. It's set to go off every few hours at random times. When the bell dings, I close my eyes, take three deep breaths through my nose, and do a general check-in with how I'm feeling in that moment. I mentally scan my body to see if I'm experiencing physical tension or emotional stress. And that's it. There's nothing else to do, nothing to fix. It's a reminder to be aware of the present moment and a way to assess if I'm spinning too fast in my day. It's been a wonderful tool to bring more calmness into my daily routine. I've been doing it for so many years that my friends and family all know about it. Whether meeting in a cafe for lunch to catch up, or at a bar over a glass of wine, or on the sofa chatting with my mom, when the mindfulness bell dings from my purse, my friends pause and close their eyes too. It takes a village to cultivate mindfulness!

Five Senses Observation

You've probably noticed the themes here: slowing down, breathing, paying attention to your body and five senses. You can do these all while sitting quietly alone or with your partner. Close your eyes, get comfortable, and take five deep breaths that fill your belly, chest, and even up to your throat, followed by a full, deep exhale. Do a general check-in with how you feel in the moment. Then, one by one, move through your five senses, spending about a minute on each one. Even though your eyes are closed, you can still check in with your sense of sight in terms of what colors, shades, and shapes you notice. Take a moment to mindfully notice all five senses at once to the best of your ability. Take a few more deep inhales and exhales and then open your eyes when you're done.

Daily Gratitudes about Your Life

One factor that repeatedly shows up in the research around the science of happiness is having a regular gratitude practice. This means being intentional every day by writing down a few things that you appreciate from the day. In the long run, you start to retrain your brain to notice more of the good in your life. I suggest a small gratitude journal by your bedside to reflect on what brought you joy, made you smile or laugh, or was delicious or interesting that day. You can also write down something that you're proud of, or something another person did that you appreciated that day. More generally, you could write about everyday things that you're taking the time to appreciate, such as a functioning car that can drive you to work, the warm sunshine, or the fact that you can get out of bed each morning. There are so many aspects to reflect on. Your gratitudes can be tiny or huge, although I encourage you always to write details about each one and reflect on *why* you feel appreciation. This kind of depth adds to the power of appreciation and increases your understanding of what makes you happy.

Positive Flip Switch[73]

Once you've been working on a daily gratitude list, start noticing which gratitudes feel the strongest to you. Stronger feelings could show up as an overall good feeling,

---

73 This concept is adapted from Lynn Grabhorn's book *Excuse Me, Your Life Is Waiting*.

a smile on your face, or a warm, expansive feeling in your heart. Each morning, choose one of these particularly "expansive" gratitudes from your ongoing nightly list and commit it to memory for the day (or write it on a note or in your phone). Then, during the day, when you notice that you're having negative thoughts that are part of a common pattern for you (e.g., I'm not good enough, I look fat, so-and-so doesn't like me), do the following four-step process:

▸ Notice the negative or self-defeating thought and label it as such.

▸ Thank the thought. I know this might sound odd, but in some way that thought is trying to help you, often by protecting you from the potential for judgment from others. Actually think or say "Thank you, thought, I appreciate that you're trying to help me, but I'm doing okay without you right now." Instead of viewing your thoughts as the enemy, you are embracing them as part of you.

▸ Choose to flip your thoughts to the powerful gratitude you chose earlier that day.

▸ Thank and congratulate yourself for noticing the negative thought and choosing to switch to something that makes you feel good.

As I said, this might sound odd, but I definitely suggest you give it a shot! Instead of beating yourself up, laugh with amusement, because there your brain goes again, having those thoughts. Then walk through the steps. This can start to break harmful cycles and thought patterns.

It's amazing to realize that we have more control over our brain chatter than we thought.

Have a Beer with Your Fear

With this cute rhyme, I don't literally mean to turn to alcohol to drown your fears. But I do suggest you approach your fears like you would an old friend, really listening to them as you would a friend while sitting at a bar and catching up. Until you gain comfort in sitting with your fears and accepting them, they will wreak havoc in the background of your life. Although they might not seem important (they're in the background, after all), your fears can actually influence your reactions, decisions, and relationships with others without you even knowing it. Pretending that fears are not there only makes this dynamic stronger and more out of your control. This feeling of being out of control often leads to behaviors that we aren't proud of.

I once heard a comparison between hiding your fears and driving a car. In this analogy, you drive in the front seat, but put your fears in the back seat. You can't see them, and you can pretend they aren't there. But as soon as something interrupts your smooth driving and you hit the brakes, your fears come flying into the front seat and splatter all over the windshield. Then you have no choice but to deal with them. You may be able to keep your feelings buried for a while, but as soon as something comes along that shakes up your normal way of moving through life, they show up in force. Unfortunately, because you're already thrown off course, these are the times that you're least equipped to handle them.

Now back to my suggestion of having a beer with your

fear. Have you ever had a difficult conversation with a friend or family member who was going through a hard time? You chose to be a source of comfort and support for them. You might have felt sad, scared, embarrassed, or disappointed—all uncomfortable emotions. But you chose to stay in that moment and be present with them, because that's what it is to be a good friend or family member. This is the same kind of nurturing and support that I'm suggesting you provide for yourself by choosing to stay in the moment with your own discomfort. Befriend your fears by accepting them exactly as they are. Once you've sat and had a few beers with them, they aren't so scary anymore.

Let's imagine that you have a fear of feeling emotionally trapped. This fear has lived in you for years, subtly influencing different areas of your life. You haven't stayed at any job for longer than two years, always worried there are better opportunities elsewhere. You tend to find flaws in your romantic partners when things become serious, as you fear making the wrong choice and being stuck with them. Rather than hating this about yourself, blaming yourself, blaming others, or ignoring this deeply ingrained fear, what if you sat and had a few beers with your fear?

You might listen to what the fear tells you about where it came from—about the first time you felt the fear and crushing weight and tightness in your chest from making the wrong decision. Your fear might suggest that it is trying to help you find the highest levels of success possible, and with success, a feeling of worthiness. Whatever your fear tells you, listen to it kindly, and thank it for trying to help you avoid pain and find happiness. Remind your fear that you've always got a choice and a voice, and that you are never truly trapped in any situation. Once you've sat and had a few beers with it, your fear may not be as scary anymore.

FORMAL PRACTICES

By formal practices, I mean setting aside time to cultivate mindfulness through more traditional activities like sitting or walking meditation, guided visualizations, or yoga. A combination of informal and formal practices aids in accelerating your mindfulness skills. The suggestions below are all activities you can do on your own, but I strongly suggest researching local or online classes in mindfulness, meditation, or compassion, because learning these practices in a community of others can support your growth.

Focus on Breathing

I wrote about taking deep breaths in the Informal Practices section, but this is an exercise with a deeper focus on breathing. Start by setting a timer for fifteen minutes, and then sit comfortably and close your eyes. Try not to regulate your breathing, but just observe it. Observe how it feels to breathe through your nose and where you feel it. Perhaps notice your chest moving up and down, or feel the air as it enters and exits your nose. Can you notice when a breath starts and when it stops? Can you feel it moving through your throat? Just observe without adding a value judgment and labeling it right or wrong. The act of concentrating on something so simple might feel quite foreign. The gaps of silence, when you are just present with the moment, may feel disconcerting at first, and you may want to move or squirm or be anywhere but sitting quietly focused on your breath. Other times, it might feel deeply relaxing and be a welcome break from the chaos of your day. Often, particularly in the beginning, it is a different experience every time you sit down to focus mindfully.

You can also choose to time two simple phrases with your in-breaths and out-breaths. This recommendation comes compliments of Thich Nhat Hanh, the Buddhist monk I quoted previously, and I learned it when I attended one of his mindfulness retreats. On the in-breath, think *present moment*, and on the out-breath, think *beautiful moment*. Present moment, beautiful moment. When I do this practice, I find it hard not to smile with the out-breath thought of *beautiful moment*.

It's likely you'll have many thoughts fighting for your attention, and that is normal and fine. When you're new to mindfulness practices, it can be helpful to identify the content of your thoughts and subsequently label them. For example, instead of focusing on your breath, you might notice you keep thinking about a deadline you have in a few hours. So you could label those thoughts "worrying" and choose to bring your focus back to your breath. Or perhaps you are making a list of the things that need to be accomplished to meet your deadline. This could be labeled "planning." Our random mind takes us all sorts of places and is much like surfing the internet. Other potentially helpful labels include "reflecting," "problem-solving," "self-berating," "berating another," "defending," "rehashing," or "remembering." Clearly labeling what's actually happening can make the flow of thoughts seem less mysterious. It gives you a way to acknowledge your thoughts and gently put them in a box as you choose to use your higher consciousness to focus on something else.

This can be particularly difficult if you believe that your thoughts in that moment are really important and you want to keep thinking about them. I know that when I'm either trying to figure out a difficult work problem or recalling a particularly pleasant experience with a man, I don't want to let go of those thoughts. One feels incredibly important and the other feels incredibly pleasurable! I literally experience this as an internal struggle when I choose to focus back on the moment. My suggestion is to remember that "mindfulness time" is best used and honored exactly as that—time to be nonjudgmentally aware and focused. You can schedule "planning time" or "worrying time" if that seems valuable to you, but do attempt to keep it separate from your mindfulness practice once you realize what's happening. Know, too, that the more you practice mindfulness, the less you'll want to let your thoughts run wild.

Guided Visualizations or Meditations

Guided visualizations or meditations involve a person facilitating your meditative experience. They may guide you through a relaxation and stress reduction activity, like imagining that you're in a peaceful location, or tensing and relaxing your body. They also might just remind you to keep coming back to your breath, or notice the sensations in your body. In general, the guides help create mental images to serve as a focal point, or verbal reminders when your mind is inevitably distracted. Our brain is a powerful tool that can create very realistic experiences, even when we're sitting quietly with our eyes closed. All such exercises create a stronger link between your mind and body and your ability to focus, thereby increasing your skills in mindfulness. Guided visualizations are a good starting point if you're new to mindfulness meditation.[74]

Loving-Kindness Meditation

A loving-kindness meditation is a specific kind of guided meditation that helps you feel more loving and kinder to yourself and others. The focus is on gratitude, compassion, and open-hearted connection. Learning how to cultivate such thoughts and emotions, and knowing what they feel like inside you, allows you to move through your everyday life in a more open and connected way. This practice makes it easier to see the good in others and helps you be more willing to reach out to friends and strangers. I mentioned the "heart center" at the end of chapter 1—this is the area around your chest where you feel deep emotions. It is common to feel warmth, contentment, and expansion in your chest during a loving-kindness meditation. It's quite a lovely feeling.

It's okay if parts of this kind of meditation feel difficult at first, as opening your heart takes practice and courage. There are many versions of loving-kindness meditation. I have a simple eight-minute version available for free on my website: www.drjennsden.com/loving-kindness-meditation.

Walking Meditation

I remember the first time I did a walking meditation while attending the retreat I referenced earlier with Thich Nhat Hanh. At 5 a.m., in the dark, dry, early morning, a group

---

74   Tara Brach has many lovely guided meditations for free here: www.tarabrach.com/guided-meditations/

of a hundred or so practitioners walked so slowly up a mountain road, we looked like zombies! It is a unique experience in mind and body connection—lifting one foot with each slow inhale and placing it gently down with each exhale. Over and over again. You can probably imagine how that pace of walking, with such focused intention on the details of lifting and placing each foot, has a rhythmic, meditative flow to it.

Another version of a walking meditation is to slowly meander through a labyrinth or nature area, consciously observing your surroundings. (This can also be done in urban settings, although that is more challenging.) I suggest you try both kinds, and notice whatever comes up in terms of thoughts, emotions, and bodily sensations. Does walking so slowly make you feel frustrated and inefficient? Great! Just observe those thoughts and feelings, without judging what you're noticing. Does walking and observing nature make you feel distracted by bugs, bright sunlight, and remembering your last camping trip? Again, great! Just notice what's coming up for you and choose to bring yourself back to observation of the present moment instead of being stuck in your brain chatter.

Yoga

While yoga classes are ubiquitous in most towns at this point, you can also get a DVD or watch a yoga class on YouTube. If you're new to yoga, I suggest attending classes before doing it on your own, so you can get direct feedback on your form. Correct form will be safer for your body, so seeking expert advice is highly recommended. But otherwise, simple home yoga practices are a fantastic way to cultivate mindfulness while moving your body.

The best kind of yoga for our purposes here is a slow-moving flow sequence, as compared to the more hardcore, high-energy yoga styles. Paying attention to your inhale and exhale, and timing your breath with your movements, has that same rhythmic flow as the slow walking meditation. Holding poses for extended periods of time, while focusing on deep breathing and your bodily sensations, can also be a full-body mindfulness practice. You may have complaints and body aches that arise the longer you hold a pose. The intent is not to torture or harm yourself, but to stand back on that shore, and kindly observe the river of mind and body chatter as it goes by.

A Word of Caution

I want to offer a word of caution about formal mindfulness practices, particularly sitting alone for meditation. If you have experienced a significant trauma and notice that those traumatic thoughts, feelings, and bodily memories come back in force when you're quietly trying to focus, I suggest you initially work with a mindfulness professional or a therapist. Having a trusted source of support is invaluable if reliving trauma is a possibility. Please don't let this scare you away from these practices, though. Doing short meditations with an external object to focus on, such as a candle, can be valuable. But do check in with your trauma and emotional resiliency so that you don't experience adverse effects while on your own.[75]

---

75 I really appreciated the discussion of this in the following article: Christopher K. Germer, "Teaching Mindfulness in Therapy," in *Mindfulness and Psychotherapy*, ed. Christopher K. Germer, Ronald D. Siegel, and Paul R. Fulton (New York: Guilford Press, 2005), 113–129.

Additionally, this is just an introduction to the vast topics of mindfulness and meditation, topics that seem to have infinite nuance and that offer unlimited insights. I highly recommend the books and work of Pema Chödrön and taking a mindfulness-based stress reduction course, both resources I've previously mentioned. Accessing resources in your local community so that you can experience, practice, and grow in a community of others is a particularly powerful path to cultivating mindfulness. I suggest an online search for mindfulness or meditation classes in your town to see whom you can connect with!

● ● ● ● ●

In an interview with Oprah, Jon Kabat-Zinn shared a profound sentence on why we would want to practice mindfulness. He said, "It's the gateway into the full dimensionality of being a human and being alive."[76] Now that you've opened this gateway, let's start applying this specifically to the interpersonal and sexual dimensions of your life.

---

76   www.oprah.com/own-super-soul-sunday/what-it-means-to-be -mindful-video

REFLECTION & WRITING

How do you think practicing mindfulness could be beneficial to you?

....
....
....
....
....

Did you have any misconceptions about what mindfulness is or isn't before reading this chapter?

....
....
....
....
....

Do you have any fears around mindfulness? If so, what are they?

....
....
....
....
....

What did you learn about your own brain that is new to you?

....
....
....
....
....

List three patterns or automatic reactions that you think the Triangle of Awareness could assist you in overcoming. (These do not have to be in the sexual realm, but could be something as simple as irritation when driving in traffic.)

1. ....
....
....

2. ....
....
....

3. ....
....
....

How might mindfulness be empowering to you?

....
....
....
....
....
....

★ ACTION ITEM ★

Find a guided visualization or meditation online and schedule time to sit quietly without interruption and follow the audio instructions. Be gentle and kind to yourself during this process.

CHAPTER 3

RELATIONSHIPS AND COMMUNICATION

The yellow sticky note on the screen door read, *Jenn may need a hug right now.*

My boyfriend chuckled when he walked through the doorway into our beach-town apartment as he returned from work one Thursday. "Does someone need a hug right now?" he called out. From the bedroom I could hear a soft laugh, as he pulled another sticky note off the living room wall. "You know I think you're beautiful, right?" he asked.

I felt my heart soften from the warmth in his voice. I knew he must have just read the note that said, *Jenn might not feel so good about her body right now.*

He sought me out in the bedroom and gave me a big, long hug. I tucked my head into his chest in embarrassment, even though nurturing was exactly what I wanted. After a few moments, I relaxed into his embrace. "Thank you," I whispered. I felt the edge of my negative mood start to wear off.

My PMS can be bad, and when I was in my twenties and early thirties, it was tough for me to voice my personal needs in the few days leading up to my period. I was often irritable, tired, and sad, with poor body image. If I didn't feel nurtured by my partner, I was more likely to unwittingly pick fights with him. This partner and I devised the sticky-note system so I could more easily ask for my needs to be satisfied, and so he knew when to give extra effort to his nurturing and his expressions of love. I created five notes, articulating different aspects of my PMS insecurities, or what I jokingly called the "shit-colored-glasses view of the world" I had for a few days each month. These notes helped me be responsible with my reactions each period cycle, even when I was emotionally struggling and lacking my usual verbal communication skills. I was grateful that my boyfriend, despite his chuckles, took the notes seriously and willingly stepped up to give me a boost of love when I was down.

• • • • •

You may have picked up this book because you struggle with intimacy in your relationships. So let's start with the word *intimacy*. What does it mean to you? Emotional closeness, trust, sharing, physical closeness, sex, being raw and real? It can mean all of these things and more. In this chapter, I primarily refer to intimacy in terms of emotional closeness, sharing, and communication. It's about being emotionally open versus being emotionally closed, and specifically, being open in communication. The most important part of intimacy is being vulnerable with someone else and receiving that vulnerability in return. You might use the word *vulnerable* to represent weakness—allowing yourself to be vulnerable to attack or to be hurt. This is one definition of the word. However, at the core of that definition, and the definition I use, is choosing to put your armor down.

When I write about vulnerability, it actually represents the opposite of weakness. To choose to be vulnerable with another person requires strength. It means feeling secure enough in yourself and with the other person to let your walls down. It's letting them see and experience the real you, in all your human beauty and messiness. And it's allowing them to do the same. This takes a lot of courage. It can be the most terrifying thing to do with another human being because of the potential of feeling judged when you've dismantled your emotional armor. Such judgment can feel like an attack on your core self. On the flip side, vulnerability is also the most beautiful and profound experience to have with another human, because there are no walls of emotional separation between you. Verbal communication at this level is profound.

Committing to this kind of vulnerability is a personal pledge to build more "conscious" relationships—that is, relationships committed to individual personal growth and also relationship growth. There are four factors most relevant in creating or maintaining a conscious relationship: vulnerability, authenticity, compassion, and mindfulness. You can probably see how the Triangle of Awareness from chapter 2 integrates all four of these: sitting with some *vulnerable* discomfort by shining a *mindful* light on your most *authentic* parts, all the while cultivating *compassion* for yourself.

Maintaining a balance among these four factors is important. For example, I worked with a married lesbian couple who were very kind to each other, and almost always compassionate and mindful about the needs of the other. This, however, worked to the detriment of their own personal needs, and they rarely held authentic and vulnerable conversations about what was not working in the marriage. This led to problems getting brushed under the rug. On the other hand, I worked with a straight couple in their thirties who enjoyed a couple glasses of wine with dinner most nights. The alcohol meant that their conversations were quite authentic and vulnerable, but the alcohol limited their capacity for mindful awareness and compassion for their partner's feelings. A balance of the four factors is invaluable, especially when communicating around uncomfortable sexual topics.

This chapter will help you apply mindfulness activities to anything that may get in the way of emotional intimacy and clear communication. You likely have fears and patterns that formed long ago, but still get triggered in your current relationships. However, you can take responsibility for your patterns, know and articulate your relationship needs, truly listen to your partner, and talk through little problems before they become big ones. In the midst of all of this, you can also focus on appreciating all the good things about your partner and relationship. You'll find that the conversations that you've been avoiding, when done through the lens of vulnerability, authenticity, compassion, and mindfulness, may actually start to bring you closer together. This chapter focuses on building skills to address overall relationship concerns and interactions; the intent is to create a stronger relationship foundation and clearer communication skills to nourish a new kind of sexual intimacy. This is what we're diving into in this chapter.

REACTIVE PATTERNS

"Mindful awareness expands our sense of self by dissolving the prison of repeating patterns of thought and response," writes Daniel Siegel.[77] One of the main things that gets in the way of honest and present communication is our reactive patterns. Early in a dating relationship, have you ever said something innocuous to your partner, only to have them unexpectedly fly off the handle? In that moment, you unwittingly triggered an uncomfortable emotion, feeling, or belief. Their angered response was indicative of an existing pattern of using anger to distance themselves from that discomfort, either by blocking it, or by stopping what's being said in that moment from continuing.

Perhaps in a similar situation, instead of lashing out in anger, your partner suddenly becomes quiet. You ask what's wrong and they say, "Nothing." Again, this is a learned pattern, probably developed long ago, to stop that discomfort. This pattern, though, is to stop discomfort by pulling back from verbal communication and retreating inward. We all have some version of these patterns. It is like a prison of the mind, and most folks don't even realize they can break out of their cell. These patterns get in the way of authentic communication and can make it difficult to create healthy, sustainable, intimate connections.

---

77   Siegel, "Mindful Awareness, Mindsight, and Neural Integration," 146.

How Expectations Create Reality

Have you ever been shopping for a specific model of car and suddenly started to notice that car everywhere you go? Your brain is trained to notice patterns. This influences what filters into your realm of observation, versus the millions of other details that you don't notice. It also influences what you *expect* to see. As previously stated, your brain operates this way because it strives for efficiency. This efficiency, though, is the opposite of mindfulness, because it creates the default of automatic pilot. Being on automatic pilot means you could miss changes in your surroundings, in your relationships, and in yourself. Change is constantly happening all around you and inside you. But these patterns cause you to unwittingly pick up your past, plop it down in the present moment, and therefore step into a future of doing the same damn things. You see and hear what you've seen and heard in your past, even when the current situation is different in so many ways.

Here is an example of a common interaction I witness with couples in my private practice. During a heated conversation about the division of chores, a woman looked from her wife to me and exclaimed, "Did you see that? She just tried to guilt me there, and make me feel bad that she usually does the dishes!" I was taken off guard, as I often am in these situations, so I honestly and gently responded, "That's not what I saw. As an outside observer, I just heard her factually state how often she does the breakfast and dinner dishes." My client paused, no longer defensive, but confused about what had happened. She had expected that I would see guilting behavior. When she was a child, her mother, who struggled with depression, had used guilt in an attempt to motivate her three children to do more chores around the house. My client expected to see guilt attached to conversations about chores, because that interpretation had been efficiently wired into her brain from a young age. Her muddied perception filtered communications in many of her relationships in this way, as it was hard for her to break that pattern. Because sexual topics tend to have even more layers of muddied assumptions, recognizing the beliefs that filter your perceptions is vital to sexual growth.

One way to make a change is to choose to stop looking for the attacks and start looking for the positive. If you look for love, kindness, listening, and affection, you will probably find more than you realized. This is a practice in being open to shifting your perspective to see what truly *is* there.[78] Positive psychology is a field of science that studies what makes humans happy and able to thrive. A lot of positive psychology research looks at how cultivating more positive perspectives improves how a person sees and experiences their world. We can influence our day-to-day happiness more than we realize by consciously cultivating positive states of mind. This doesn't mean you're ignoring bad stuff; it just means you're intentionally looking for the good stuff.

Another aspect of taking responsibility for your emotions and shifting your pattern of expectations is being able to recognize the signs that you're getting overwhelmed in any given moment. When you're over-

---

78   This section was adapted from my blog post "Did You Miss the Moonwalking Bear? How Expectations Create Our Reality," posted on January 12, 2012: www.drjennsden.com/blog/2012/1/12/did-you-miss-the-moonwalking-bear-how-expectations-create-ou.html

whelmed, negative emotions become too strong, and you lose access to your higher cognitive functions. It's important to catch it *when* it's happening, before you cross a line and say or do things you later regret. This is where mindful awareness of your bodily sensations is an incredibly helpful tool, because you can notice where and when you're feeling warm, tingly, tense, or restless.

I had a forty-nine-year-old client who noticed that when he was becoming angry and getting close to losing control of his temper, his ears would feel warm and there would be a growing prickly feeling on the back of his neck. Another client, a thirty-nine-year-old man, observed what he called a "buzzy feeling" in his head when he was feeling emotionally flooded. They were able to use these bodily sensations as warning signs to step away from the situation. I instructed them to explain all of this to their partners ahead of time, along with the out-of-control consequences they were hoping to avoid. Then, I urged them to calmly and responsibly ask for space to move away and cool down when they noticed those sensations, then return to the conversation twenty minutes later (or after more time, if needed) with fresh eyes and calmer emotions.

Conflict Resolution

It is very common for resentments to slowly build in a relationship until they take on a life of their own, so here is another powerful tool for communicating about your triggers and resentments in your relationship. I call it the Conflict Resolution Tool or the Healthy Resentments Process. Although anything can create a resentment (I know a woman who would get incredibly irritated by how her partner chewed), this process is intended for topics that are difficult to move on from.

In general, you will use this communication technique at some point after you've felt hurt or angry with your partner, or after the two of you have had a conflict that hasn't been resolved. You should only use this process regarding a specific problematic situation, and not for general grievances (e.g., use it for the incident the other night in the car coming home from the restaurant, not for an ongoing complaint about how you never feel heard). As with anything done mindfully, this is about taking responsibility for what's showing up for you, instead of blaming it on someone else. Here are the steps:

1. Permission. Ask your partner permission to share something that's been on your mind and to use this process. This is a much more respectful approach than just launching into a topic that your partner might not be ready to handle responsibly. (If you are the person on the receiving end of this permission request, it is your responsibility to do a self-check and make sure you're not distracted, hungry, or irritable, and that you can bring the best you've got to this interaction. If the timing isn't right for you, counteroffer with another time within the next twenty-four hours. Once you agree on another time, it's your responsibility to put it in your calendar and approach your partner at the appointed time to have this discussion. Don't assume your partner will bring up the topic again— take on that responsibility yourself.)

2. Facts. Once you're having the discussion, start by sharing the facts of the situation that upset you. Share the context you were in, who was there, the time of day, whether you'd eaten recently, what was said (as close to verbatim as you can remember), and anything else that is relevant. You and your partner get to agree on the facts of the situation and make sure that interpretations aren't being misconstrued as facts. For example, a fact would be: "It was 11 p.m., we had each had three drinks in two hours, and you said that we had not had sex in six months. Then we didn't talk for the next twenty minutes until we left the bar." A non-factual, subjective statement would be: "It was late and you were drunk and being mean to me."

3. Interpretations. This is when you get to share your interpretations of what happened. What did it mean to you? What did it remind you of? For example, did it remind you of when an ex used to talk to you in a condescending way? Just like with the Thoughts part of the Triangle, you're stating that you recognize this as your reality, not a statement of fact or indication of your partner's intent. Use statements like: "My interpretation was . . ." and "I know this might not be what you intended, but what it meant to me was . . ." Your partner should be silent while listening to you share your interpretations (presuming you are being verbally responsible in your ownership of your interpretations). To build on the facts presented above, an example of this could be, "When you said that we hadn't had sex in six months, I thought that you were trying to make me feel bad. I was thinking about all the stress that I've had at work in the last six months, and I thought it was selfish of you to ask for sex. My interpretation was that you were trying to make me feel guilty. Then I thought you were disappointed with me."

4. Emotions. What were you feeling? Fear, embarrassment, shame, disappointment, abandonment, anxiety, sadness, anger? Be mindful to say "I felt . . ." instead of "You made me feel . . ." As a reminder, if your main emotion was anger, frustration, or irritation, take your self-reflection deeper and see what is beneath that anger, if anything. Feel free also to share *where* in your body you felt or still feel those emotions. During this sharing of emotions, your partner remains silent and attentively listens to you. For example, you might say, "When you said that we hadn't had sex in six months, I felt defensive and pissed at first. Then I felt overwhelmed and worried. And then my heart started pounding because I was scared you might want to end the relationship." Writing down what you want to say in steps two to four ahead of time can help you articulate your concerns.

5. Request. This last step isn't always necessary, but the intent is to give you a space to make a concrete request for your partner to say or do something differently in the future. In the story at the beginning of the chapter, I had negotiated with my boyfriend and made the specific request that he hug and compliment me more during my PMS each month. This request served both of us, since we were much less likely to fight when I felt a boost of nurturing and love during these times. Your partner has the right to negotiate with you until you both agree on a concrete step to try to sidestep this conflict in the future. To conclude the above example, you could make the following request: "Can we schedule an evening out in the next week so that we can have some adult conversation and quality time? I think I would be more interested in sex then." Or you could request, "Could we please not bring up the sex topic when we're drinking? I think we both need to be on top of our mindfulness skills to discuss a sensitive topic like that."[79]

Articulating your concerns and needs in this way will take time to learn, and I suggest that you mark these pages and take notes or make a photocopy or take a picture of the steps, so you can both honor the integrity of this process. While it may feel formal and awkward at first, don't let that stop you from becoming more comfortable with each step in the way it is described. Over time, once you feel more competent with the skill of speaking your truth this way, you can make it your own. But don't let a fear of feeling awkward get in the way of committing yourself to this valuable process—addressing resentments is when you want to consciously cultivate your brave energy!

The Gift of Presence

During a free-flowing conversation with your partner, it can be easy to interrupt them and not even realize that this is a reactive pattern. Staying present during a conversation can be a challenge because you may be distracted by other thoughts, bored, or preparing what to say next. Added to this is the familiarity of being in a conversation with your loved one, a person who also pushes your buttons. You know them so well, you sometimes assume you know what they're going to say before they say it. You might be irritated with the direction you think the conversation

---

79   The process I present here is loosely based on Marshall B. Rosenberg's four-step nonviolent communication process.

is going, so you interrupt. For all these reasons and more, staying truly present, listening, and being aware of the person in front of you while they're talking can be tough, but it is monumental for effective communication.

I would argue that being present for someone, as a witness to their words and emotions, is one of the biggest gifts we can give another person. Plus, it's free! It's interesting that the word "present" means both being in the moment and giving a gift. In this case, it means both simultaneously. Mindful listening is a gift to your partner. Shining the light of your undivided attention on your partner shows respect, acknowledgment, and love.

A good way to build this skill is by doing a regular practice in attentive listening with your partner. In this case, attentive listening is listening to your partner speak with the intent to understand the meaning of their sharing and why it matters to them to speak about this topic. The simplest way to do this is to decide on an amount of time (e.g., three or five minutes) that you each want to talk and flip a coin to determine who goes first. Then set a timer as the first person shares about their day, or whatever is on their mind (but don't choose a hot topic for you two). The second person just listens with rapt attention. The listener can react with facial expressions that mirror what their partner is feeling or the tone of the topic (e.g., smile, laugh, nod, express worry), but they should not speak. Remember, this is about the person sharing, not about the listener.

If, while participating in this exercise, you notice that you feel frustrated or irritated by not speaking or by what your partner is saying, do not judge those emotions, but do observe where you feel those emotions in your body.

With a few in-breaths, visually imagine your breath going to those areas of your body. This can help you stay present with those uncomfortable sensations and also bring some relaxation to your body. Then choose to bring your attention back to your partner. Once the timer goes off, you are free to ask a few clarifying questions to better understand. If your partner shared about a challenging situation, don't use this time to try to "fix" that, such as telling them a way they could have reacted or handled the situation differently Then switch roles. Through mindful listening over time, you'll learn more nuances about what matters to your partner and how they communicate their needs. You'll also likely feel heard and understood by your partner to a degree that is new and welcome.

Taking Responsibility for Your Triggers and Needs

One of the most common patterns in intimate relation-ships is to blame your partner, but as I often tell my clients, it takes two to tango. This means that you both have a role and responsibility in almost every issue that arises, even when you are sure you're blameless. Even if a conflict situation is clearly caused by your partner's reactivities, insecurities, or problematic patterns, if you're choosing to be in a partnership with them (and, presumably, believe it is a healthy and beneficial relationship), then I believe you also have a responsibility to make different choices in this conflict.

Think about the difference between the words "blame" and "responsibility." The energy behind blame is one of negativity, heaviness, righteousness, and stagnation. Responsibility, on the other hand, feels lighter and more optimistic, and has a potential for positive change. These distinctions can make a big difference when struggling with difficult relationship topics. It might also help to remember that some of our triggers come from the unhealthy societal messages that surround us. For example, think of any mainstream romantic comedy movie; most likely there was a time when the woman felt jealous and lashed out, when she obsessed about what to wear, and when she had sex and quickly experienced an orgasm. The overall message is probably that despite her success in life, she's not really fulfilled and complete without the perfect man. These messages create the madness that limits women's self-worth and sexual expression, and they can certainly affect the way women view their own triggers. If we take responsibility for making changes and overcoming these messages, instead of blaming ourselves or others, we can move forward in relationship growth.

I once coached a young woman for several years, and then transitioned into coaching her and her new boyfriend together. They were struggling with some of her reactive patterns around her expectations of him. If she was sharing a work story about a disrespectful interaction that day, a situation that was particularly agitating to her, he felt bad that work had upset her and wanted her to feel better. Sometimes he would immediately troubleshoot the problem and try to fix it. Other times he would listen but not exhibit any emotions. His ways of responding were creating more agitation for her, and that would lead to arguments. They recognized that this was a pattern, and both were willing to take responsibility and to step up and try something new.

I asked if he was aware of this pattern in the moment, and he said yes. Whenever she was in emotional pain, he would notice that he felt stuck and unsure of what to say next. Then he would hear her growing anger and freeze even more. Feeling emotionally stuck when in a difficult conversation had been a familiar feeling to him his entire life. I suggested that when this happened, he switch gears by acknowledging to her that he's not responding in the way she would like, and then asking her two questions: 1) "What could I have said differently?" and 2) "Why is it important to you that I say that in this situation?"

These questions would help her see that he was trying to support her, and they would also turn the responsibility back on her to identify what she really needed in that moment. The second question would help them bridge the gap between their different interpretations of what was going on, because it asked for the *meaning* of the situation to her. This question would get to the heart of what she really needed and wanted in the moment. In this case, we uncovered that what she most needed was to hear him empathize with how unfair her boss was and to recognize that she felt embarrassed. It mattered to her that he say those things, because to her, that meant her emotional struggles were valid.

On her side, she had the responsibility to recognize that he couldn't read her mind, and to own her irritated reactions to him for not knowing the right way to support her. She also had the responsibility of acknowledging, with patience, when he was mindfully trying to do things differently. I suggested that after answering his two questions, she ask in return: "Does this have the same or different meaning to you now?" Again, this would help them bridge the gap between their differing interpretations. There are a lot of moving parts to a situation like this, but when both partners are willing to be responsible, mindful, and compassionate, it's possible to change these deep patterns.

We often don't ask directly and clearly for what we need in our close relationships. Logically, it seems obvious—if we need something, just ask for it. So how did it become so complicated for so many people? Why is it that a direct, honest approach doesn't seem easy, appropriate, or even like an option? See if one of the five statements below resonates with you:

> I think it is pathetic to have to request what I need.
> I can take care of myself, and don't need to ask for help.
> It's selfish to request my needs, and it's an imposition on my partner.
> If my partner really loved me, they would be able to anticipate or already know my needs.
> I don't know how to ask for my needs in a way that doesn't seem controlling or demanding.

These are common beliefs I hear expressed by everyone. The first three beliefs often stem from a similar childhood experience: You learned that your needs didn't matter. Did you learn from a young age that your needs weren't going to be met? Were you ridiculed when you expressed your vulnerability and asked for something? Were you told to be seen and not heard? Were you not allowed to express your needs? Or perhaps your family was struggling in some way, whether financially, with mental illness, or addiction, and the needs of your parents or siblings seemed more important than your own? If you experienced any of these regularly as a kid, it makes perfect sense that you wouldn't be comfortable or skilled in requesting your needs as an adult.

The fourth belief, on the other hand, is based on romanticized notions of what love is, and the idea that your partner should be able to read your mind. Frankly, while that romantic notion is often depicted in books and movies, it's incredibly unfair to your partner and generally impossible. The fifth belief is often the result of being new to requesting your needs, and needing time and practice to be calm, fair, and compassionate when doing so.

One of the tools I love using with couples is the book *The 5 Love Languages* and the free online thirty-question quiz.[80] This book by Gary Chapman is based on the idea that there are five basic ways we can give or receive love, and that we are all wired differently around how we want to be loved. The five "languages" are quality time, physical touch, gifts, words of affirmation, and acts of service. You might feel like you're showing love and caring for your partner by making meals, doing laundry, and cleaning up (i.e., acts of service), but your partner might feel most loved and connected when trying a new restaurant together while you each talk about your day (i.e., quality time). Or, when you're upset, your partner might want to touch you and hold you to show love and support (i.e., physical touch), but that might feel awkward because you just want to hear that they love and believe in you (i.e., words of affirmation).

I see couples "loving past each other" in this way all the

---

time in my private practice. It's clear to me that they love each other, but they don't feel it in a meaningful way from their partner, and their partner feels unappreciated for all that they *do* do. This is why I think the term "language" is so appropriate—the style of love your partner wants and needs from you might feel foreign and uncomfortable, just like learning a new language. Becoming fluent in your partner's love language often requires new knowledge, genuine effort, kind feedback, and patience on both sides. By taking and applying the *The 5 Love Languages* quiz, you can take responsibility for learning to voice your needs in new ways, and also for filling your partner's love bucket in meaningful ways.

For example, let's say your partner goes out with his friends on your one night off, so you give him the silent treatment in bed when he comes home that night. You're pissed because you think he's wasting time with his friends. Beneath that anger are hurt feelings and disappointment, because quality time together is how you best connect and feel loved, but he seems to be prioritizing time with his friends. Your partner, on the other hand, doesn't understand your reaction because quality time is not one of his top love languages. He gets upset that you didn't appreciate all the acts of service (his top love language) he did for you, like leaving you dinner in the fridge, cleaning the apartment, and texting you when he was coming home. Identifying your underlying love language need and speaking from that place is vulnerable, but this is how you can actually move the conversation forward, instead of getting stuck in ongoing arguments. Responsibly requesting to have your quality-time need addressed could look like asking for a special Friday night date night, or scheduling a midweek lunch together at a new restaurant. It's okay to gently remind your partner how you feel most loved and connected.

I have another suggestion for a really lovely way to get clearer on what is most important to each of you in your partnership. Get some paper and pens and sit down quietly together to each answer the following six questions:

> ▸ I feel most in love with you when . . .
> ▸ I like you the most when . . .
> ▸ I'm most proud of you when . . .
> ▸ I feel most intimate with you when . . .
> ▸ I feel most nurtured by you when . . .
> ▸ I wish every day we could . . .

Approach these questions from a positive perspective. For example, you could write, "I like you the most when you're doing something that you're passionate about, and you express that happiness to me." On the other hand, a negative answer to that question, or a backhanded way of approaching it, might be, "I like you the most when you're not nagging me about doing chores around the house." I'm sure you can see how the first response is helpful and loving and the second one is snippy and negative. Other than that, there is no right or wrong way to answer these questions, and it's fine to expand on your answers if you feel inspired by what your partner shares.

SMALL HURTS VERSUS BIG HURTS

It stings when you feel hurt by your partner. Sometimes, though, it can feel even worse when you're the one who does the hurting—when you hurt your partner's feelings. Part of the socialization of the "good girl" ideology is to place the needs of others first, especially a male partner. But it is impossible to avoid differences in beliefs, needs, desires, and priorities in a relationship. You are two separate people with distinctive genetic predispositions and different upbringings. You're going to have discrepancies in needs, values, and expectations. A problem arises, though, when you continually bury your needs to avoid conflict, hurting their feelings, or disappointing them. Frankly, occasionally disappointing and hurting your partner is a healthy and necessary part of any relationship.

Your partner might have this same kind of avoidance pattern. If your partner is male, he may have been raised with the belief that he should never hurt a woman. For many men, seeing the woman they love cry because of something that they did or said is an intensely uncomfortable experience. They feel responsible for her pain and powerless to make it stop. If you and your partner are both avoiding hurting the other, eventually the pile of junk brushed under the rug becomes so large that you can't help but trip over these relationship resentments. Once you're getting to the point of tripping over them, it means those small hurts have now become big hurts. So what can you do to nip this in the bud?

It should come as no surprise that my answer is to try mindfulness. If you're avoiding conflict, the discomfort of addressing a concern head-on is greater than the discomfort of suppressing your needs. So figure out what is so uncomfortable about addressing that concern. This may include a desire to avoid hurting your partner, embarrassment, shame, or even pride. Once you've figured out why you're avoiding the conflict, you'll be better prepared to address the conflict itself.

I once worked with a heterosexual married couple in their late forties. The husband was a gregarious storyteller, and they hosted many late-night parties with live music and laughter. She had a quieter demeanor but enjoyed hosting parties as well. As the parties would wind down, it was common to have a small group of friends gathered around a table as the conversation turned to politics or social issues. The wife would share an insightful comment about an article she had read, but the conversation would continue on, her statement unacknowledged. Five minutes later, her husband would share the same insightful comment, but he would be met with praise and acknowledgement. For many years, the wife internalized her resentment, not wanting to rock the boat or cause discomfort for her husband. She knew he didn't even realize it was happening. But over time, she resented his male privilege and lack of awareness. This small hurt had become a big hurt, with much greater baggage to unpack.

When I used the Triangle with her, we learned that she was embarrassed in these situations, feeling visceral discomfort in her chest and solar plexus. She believed she was perceived as less intelligent than her husband, and she felt a constriction in her throat—she was literally silenced—because her words didn't seem to matter. She also believed that he didn't care about this happening because he enjoyed the attention and praise. When we examined why she had avoided telling her husband about this, she realized she didn't want to hurt his feelings or create an awkward social situation, so she never said anything.

Her husband was shocked to learn how much this hurt her, and while he did like the attention, he didn't want his needs fulfilled at the expense of her voice and self-esteem. They began approaching these situations as a team. She reminded him before parties to pay attention to this dynamic, and he called it out in the group when he noticed. Other times, because she knew she had his support, she felt confident enough to point out these occurrences, and he backed her up. Although the pattern didn't go away, they were now working mindfully together to address it, and she wasn't further disempowered.

Are there specific times when you suppress your needs for your partner? This isn't necessarily a bad thing, as we all need to compromise in relationships. But if you are building resentment each time and not responsibly voicing that resentment, then you've got a problem. Do you go along with your partner's parenting discipline style, despite cringing inside? Have you faithfully been accompanying your partner to church each week, but resenting the messages you are exposed to? Are you saying yes to unwanted sex, grinning and bearing through the pain until he comes? All of these circumstances warrant a mindful conversation. These will be uncomfortable conversations, for sure. But if you want your relationship to have the potential to thrive in the long run, you need to address these smaller issues when they surface in the short term.

GRATITUDES AND ACKNOWLEDGMENTS

When you've been in a relationship for a while, it's easy to focus more on the negative than on the positive. In the beginning when you really like someone, the surprises and newness, as well as the positive neurochemicals, create a short-term positivity haze. However, in a long-term relationship, it's easy to emphasize the opposite. So it's not unusual in long-term relationships to notice more of the negative things than the positive. When you're focusing on the priorities of maintaining a household, balancing your relationship and work, raising children, or going to school, it makes sense that you're going to notice what is not running smoothly. Some researchers argue that this "negativity bias" is actually genetically influenced. As a survival mechanism, we are programmed to notice what is wrong or not working, just like other animals. Not surprisingly, this negativity bias can be a real downer in a relationship if every day you're hit with a litany of complaints.

If this resonates with you, I suggest making a conscious shift from being in a relationship that is based on surviving to a relationship that is based in thriving. Break through the negativity bias by shifting to a strengths-based approach and consciously focusing on what you like and what is working. Optimism is a choice; the foundation of your relationship is much stronger when you both commit to cultivating it. Below are several practices to integrate more verbal appreciation into your relationship.

I want to be clear that these activities are intended for healthy and respectful relationships. If your partner is physically or emotionally abusive, please do not focus on the positive by brushing the abuse under the rug. (If you think you might be in an abusive relationship, call the National Domestic Violence Hotline for confidential help at any hour, at 1-800-799-7233.)

Daily Gratitudes

Relationship researcher John Gottman argues that a 5:1 balance of positive to negative comments and interactions is the ideal in a lasting relationship.[81] One way to improve this ratio is a daily commitment to share one or two things you appreciate about your partner that day. For example, do you like the way the color of their shirt brings out the color of their eyes, the way they handled a difficult situation with your child, that they remembered to clean the morning dishes, or their creativity in repairing a broken object? If you look hard enough, the list is endless. Include details about what you appreciated or why you're expressing gratitude for that thing. It's one thing to say, "You look nice today." It's a totally different thing to say, "I love how your suit accentuates your build and shows off how much you've been working out recently." If you're away from each other, you can still text or email a couple of qualities that you admire in them or a favorite memory from the past. Ideally, you and your partner will make expressing gratitude a regular part of your daily interactions, and this structured approach is a great way to create this habit.

---

81   This is a great short article from The Gottman Institute about creating the 5:1 ratio: www.gottman.com/blog/the-magic-relationship-ratio-according-science

Celebrating Successes

Making and taking time to celebrate when something good has happened, even if it's relatively small, is often overlooked in relationships. How often do you take the time to celebrate what is working, and to celebrate the happy things that happen to each of you as individuals in your work, parenting, friendships, exercise, etc.? Are you the first person your partner wants to share exciting news with because they appreciate your positive and supportive reactions? Are they the first person you want to share with, because they make the good news feel even better? The best of these kinds of enthusiastic interactions are when you not only celebrate your partner's good news with positive feedback, but also compliment them and focus on the positive aspects of the event.

Martin Seligman, positive psychologist and author of *Flourish*, uses the example of receiving a promotion and sharing that good news with your partner. An active and constructive way for your partner to respond to that news is to congratulate you and tell you how proud they are, ask for details about how you found out, and ask how you two could celebrate, all the while smiling and maintaining eye contact. At the other end of the spectrum, your partner could focus on the potential negative aspects of that news, asking if you'll be away from the family more, expressing worry, or simply not reacting and saying something unrelated.[82] That would feel deflating, no? Check in every day in your relationship and ask whether there is any success, small or large, to be celebrated.

---

82   Martin E. P. Seligman, *Flourish: A Visionary New Understanding of Happiness and Well-Being* (New York: Simon & Schuster, 2011), 49.

Fifteen Things I Love About You

One of my favorite suggestions for a free yet extremely meaningful Valentine's Day or birthday present is to write a list of at least fifteen things you appreciate about your partner. What are their gifts? Positive traits? Which characteristics first grabbed your heart? If you both take the time to do this, you can share your lists with each other, then post them in a place where you will see them often. As I mentioned previously, including details about why you like that specific thing makes this process much more powerful for both of you. Try to *feel* the heart expansion of appreciation when you write these. The following are a handful of appreciation categories to assist in writing your list. These can also be used with your daily gratitudes to each other (see page 131).

How they nurture you. Does your partner know just the right thing to do when you're stressed? Do they take care of you when you're sick, setting you up on the sofa with a cup of hot tea, the remote, and a warm blanket? Do they offer insightful feedback on your blog posts before you post them? We all feel nurtured by different things, from having a meal prepared for you, to having your clothes folded in a particular way, having your car washed, or being treated to a meal or a soothing foot massage. What does your partner do that makes you feel safe and grounded and important?

The traits you fell in love with. Can your partner make you laugh, even when you're mad at them? Are they so kind to stray animals that it makes your heart ache? Are they more sexually comfortable and adventurous than you, and willing to gently bring new ideas to the bedroom? Hopefully you have a long list of traits that first attracted you to your partner, and that still impress you.

What you have in common. Do you like to read the same mystery novels and discuss their plots? Is a Sunday morning hike your shared idea of a perfect weekend activity? Do you like to hit up farmers' markets and try cooking new meals together? Perhaps you both like to de-stress from your day by watching the same Netflix series. Write down some of your favorite shared hobbies and how you feel when you get to enjoy them together.

Favorite memories. Remember that trip to the Grand Canyon when you forgot to pack the tent and you ended up staying in the most romantic Airbnb ever? Or the shared beauty and awe of your first ocean sunset, being at the top of the Eiffel Tower, or the birth of your first child? Maybe you got so drunk one night, you skinny-dipped in your neighbor's pool. Whether the memory evokes awe, appreciation, or laughter, share a few that move you the most.

Shared values. Do you both like to squirrel away money to save for a big family vacation to your favorite amusement park? Are your political values aligned? Do you both donate to the same nonprofits? Do you share the same values in how to raise your children? Consider the values that you have in common that create stability in your relationship and life goals.

How they make you a better version of you. Does your partner notice when you're getting frustrated with your son and jump in to give you a break? Will they meditate with you each morning because that's an important routine for you, or give you yoga class gift cards for your birthday because they know that's your happy place? Maybe they've supported your family financially so you could finish your college degree. The best relationships create a synergy that encourages continual growth and a desire to be better people.

Because you are providing details, your partner will likely learn new things about what they mean to you. While fifteen items might seem like a lot at first, these categories will likely prime you to see that there are so many reasons to love and appreciate your partner. Again, give yourself the time and space to really *feel* these appreciations as you write down the details.[83]

Weekly Acknowledgments

So far, all of these gratitude and strengths-related activities have involved you sharing what you like about your partner and vice versa. This Weekly Acknowledgements process, though, turns that on its head. Instead of offering what you appreciate, you first ask your partner what they would like to be appreciated for. The intent of this activity is to ensure that you both feel appreciated for what you're contributing and accomplishing in your relationship and life, and to learn what matters to your partner in this realm.

When I introduce this to a couple in a coaching session, it's common for one or both to end up with tears down

---

83   This section was adapted from my article "15 Things I Love About You," first published on The Good Men Project on February 8, 2014: goodmenproject.com/featured-content/15-things-love-bmartin

their faces. It feels really good to them to feel appreciated in the eyes of their partner, specifically for the strengths and accomplishments that they feel proud of. Sharing what you'd like to be acknowledged for does not mean that you did that activity because you wanted praise. It is a way of saying, "I did something good," and then allowing your partner to know that and acknowledge you for it. Here are five steps to guide this process for you:

▸ Ask your partner what they have done in the past week that they would like to be acknowledged for. They should share what they think they have done well, whether it is accomplishments, positive interactions, improvements, household contributions, going out of their way for someone, being kind to an animal, remembering something they usually forget, changing a behavior, being a good listener, exercising, being patient, etc. Your partner should aim to name at least three things. (I suggest making at least one of them about something specific to your relationship.)

▸ Once your partner has articulated what they want acknowledgement for, say, "[Partner's name], I would like to acknowledge you for . . ." and repeat in your own words what they have said. Also add in anything else around those topics that is meaningful to you, or anything else from the past week that you appreciate them for.

▸ Switch roles and do it again.

It may feel awkward at first to ask for what you want to be praised for, and for the other person to actually say, "I want to acknowledge you for such-and-such." But it can also be really beneficial if you give it a chance. First, it allows you to receive appreciation for what you're happy about. Second, hearing praise from someone else's mouth, *even when you asked for it*, can feel nourishing and grounding. Third, realizing what your partner wants to be praised for makes it easier to understand them and to better appreciate their attributes. Fourth, by including additional praise along the way, your partner can hear how you view their accomplishments, and they can bask in the glory of your admiration. When this process starts to feel more natural, it becomes easier to integrate acknowledgments into everyday interactions, which overall increases the positive energy in the relationship. Being able to ask for and articulate praise is a great step towards focusing on the positive, improving understanding, and increasing intimacy. Feel free to specifically ask for acknowledgments from your sexual interactions as well![84]

All of these activities can help uncover what you love about your partner and prompt you to be more likely to give them the benefit of the doubt when you are having difficult conversations. Remember that the negativity bias is built into us as humans, but with greater awareness and presence, we can retrain our brains. A daily commitment to these kinds of activities imbues a positivity bias to your relationship. The benefits are many, including

---

84   I learned this general concept of acknowledgments through the Accomplishment Coaching training program in San Diego, when I was their "demonstration client" in 2004–2005: www .accomplishmentcoaching.com

appreciating your partner's strengths, seeing all the ways they contribute that you take for granted, feeling appreciated in all that you provide, and creating a buffer for the tough times. Regularly practicing gratitude helps you realize the goodwill of your partner, be more open-minded to creative solutions, and give each other space to mess up yet keep moving forward. This foundation is so important as we move into the next chapter and specifically address sexual communication and desire.

REFLECTION & WRITING

What patterns or triggers do you think you have in relationships? List three of them below, and for each, identify when or how you think it started and the accompanying thoughts, emotions, and bodily sensations. Can you actually feel where each one lives inside you?

1. ....
....
....
....
....
....
....

2. ....
....
....
....
....
....
....

3. ....
....
....
....
....
....
....

Write down three to five things you need to feel happy and supported in a relationship. Is it hard for you to identify your needs in a relationship? Are you able to responsibly voice your needs to your partner? How might you be able to start responsibly requesting your needs?

1. ....
....
....
....

2. ....
....
....
....

3. ....
....
....
....

4. ....
....
....
....
....

5. ....
....
....
....
....

What are your biggest strengths regarding healthy communication in your relationship, or in past relationships?

....

....

....

....

....

....

....

....

What do you think are your biggest areas for improvement regarding communication in your relationship, or in past relationships?

....

....

....

....

....

....

....

....

★ ACTION ITEM ★

Contact your partner right now and share three things you really appreciate about them. If you are single, write an "I love me because . . ." note to yourself with at least three strengths or accomplishments of which you are proud.

CHAPTER 4

SEX, PASSION, AND DESIRE

The grass tickled my forearms as I cupped my head with my clasped hands. The scratchy picnic blanket wasn't big enough for both of us to lie down without our limbs spilling onto the lawn. I willed myself to take a few deep breaths as I tried to focus on the slow-moving puffy clouds overhead. The tightness in my chest felt like an iron ball of hot anger.

"Wait. So you're saying that we *both* have to *work* on this?" my boyfriend asked in shock.

Every nerve in my body wanted to explode. It was a good thing we were at Central Park in New York City, with a lot of innocent tourists wandering around. "Yes," I said through clenched teeth. "I've been telling you that since our first kiss." That kiss had been almost two and a half years earlier.

"I know you said that you tend to lose your desire after a couple years in a relationship, but since that's your specialty area at work, I thought you'd just take care of it on your own and fix it," he blurted out.

Was he kidding? Thoughts were swirling in my head and I clenched my jaw to keep them from escaping my lips. *I was so conscientious and proactive in telling him about my low desire in long-term relationships, so how did that backfire on me? How does he not realize that it takes two people to make a sex life work? How does he not want to work on this?* The last thought evoked flutters of anxiety in my chest, replacing some of the fiery anger. I sat up with restless energy and turned my back to him. I watched an older couple walk by with matching sunburned necks.

"So you thought that the passion and ease of sex at the beginning of our relationship would last? Even though I told you repeatedly that from my end it wouldn't?" I asked.

"Uh, yeah," he said.

"And so that's why every time I want to sit down and create a plan so we can address our waning sex life, and try to do something different, you're not willing to do anything?"

"I don't *want* to do anything differently. I want sex like we had in the beginning," he barked. "You're saying all of that in the beginning was a lie? It wasn't real?" Now he was stammering.

"No. That was real. It was definitely real. I wasn't faking my interest and passion. But this, now, is also real," I sighed. I felt my heart sink into my stomach. Clearly this topic was not going to be cleared up during our afternoon picnic in the park.

●　●　●　●　●

Sexual passion and desire can seem easy to experience . . . until they're not anymore. In general, we are ill equipped to handle any kind of sexual problems that arise. When our desire is more naturally present at the beginning of a relationship, we go with the flow and don't think about it. But as time goes on, and we remain with the same partner, it's not uncommon for women to experience a drop in physiological desire. If we expect to have sex like twenty-year-olds, or as we did at the start of a new relationship, for our entire lives, we'll be sorely disappointed. We'll also be missing out on a lot.

Many women like and enjoy sex as much as many men do. Women can be just as horny as men, or more. There's a funny assumption around sex, though, that I think we learn from Hollywood movies and romance novels: If two people really love each other, then sex and desire should be easy, spontaneous, and always available. This is just not factual. I do believe that once the romantic phase of dating has passed in heterosexual relationships, women often have lower sexual desire than men in their relationships. I've seen this repeatedly in my private practice, and there is growing research to support it.[85] While there are numerous environmental factors for this, most of which are the focus of this book, it's valuable to also consider relevant biological and physiological factors. Some women (just like some men) naturally have a lower level of sexual desire, and some women experience a noticeable drop in desire after a certain point in dating (often anywhere from eight months to three years). There are

---

85   Annika Gunst et al., "Female Sexual Function Varies over Time and Is Dependent on Partner-Specific Factors: A Population-Based Longitudinal Analysis of Six Sexual Function Domains," *Psychological Medicine* 47, no. 2 (2016): 341–352, doi:10.1017/s0033291716002488

absolutely men who fall into these categories as well, but statistically, it is more likely for women to experience this shift. And it's common for everyone to experience wide changes in sexual desire over a lifetime.

The number-one reason why a woman visits a sex therapist or counselor is because she feels that her sexual desire is too low in her relationship. The phrasing "in her relationship" is relevant because it is the relationship context that matters, for two reasons: One, because it is often within a relationship that has moved beyond the early lustful, romantic phase that she doesn't feel her passion as much, and two, because within her relationship her desire level is being compared to that of her partner (her male partner, if she's in a heterosexual relationship, but perhaps still to male sexuality overall even if she's in a same-sex relationship). Most people experience changing levels of desire throughout their lives based on their health, relationships, and other factors, and when a woman experiences this drop, she may view herself as broken in some way.

I've seen this scenario so many times in my private practice: The couple had a sexual connection in the beginning of the relationship, but after a few years, or after having children, the woman doesn't feel like having sex anymore. She still loves and respects her partner, but her body is no longer asking for sex. I have also worked with couples in which the man experiences a drop in desire and passion, and the woman is the one who misses their sexual connection. And I've also worked with lesbian couples in which one woman still desires sexual intimacy and the other woman has lost her appetite. Any time there is a drop in sexual desire from one partner but not the other, it can put a strain on the relationship.

This scenario usually plays out with the partner with the higher sex drive feeling rejected, unloved, unwanted, or physically unattractive. Let's say it's a man, who wants to feel desired and connect deeply with his partner through sexual activity, but that isn't happening anymore. Or the couple may be having obligatory sex, but he really wants her to feel and express passion, and he wants to know that she's enjoying herself. On the flip side, the woman feels guilty or broken. She may get irritated by his sexual advances, but deep down is feeling inadequate that she can't give him what he wants anymore. This can lead to deep hurt and resentments on both sides. Often this disparity in desire becomes the elephant in the room that does not get discussed or addressed responsibly. Our romantic notions of love lead us to believe that the excitement and passion felt in the short term will be the same in a long-term, committed, stable, loving relationship. Unfortunately, this expectation and the subsequent shift in desire levels sets up many couples for disappointment and disconnection.[86]

This chapter explores the complexity of sexual desire and women's ability to enjoy the pleasures associated with sexual activity. I explore issues ranging from why you may want to avoid sexual conversations and how to move through that resistance, to the blocks that might thwart sexual desire and how to start overcoming them. You'll have a lot to reflect on by the end of the chapter. As you work your way through this chapter, consider how what you've read in earlier chapters applies to what you're reading here.

---

86   Author Esther Perel has published a wonderful book, titled *Mating in Captivity*, on this topic.

WHAT DOES SEX MEAN TO YOU?

Sex is a complicated topic. It's presented in the media as a simple, straightforward concept and activity, but as you've been reading in this book and probably already know innately, it has a lot of components. As a society and as individuals, we make sex mean many different things. We often assume that what it means to us is just what's normal for everyone. But humans are more varied than we think in what meanings we attach to sex, and therefore how we experience it.

A fantastic research study at the University of Texas at Austin analyzed why college students have sex.[87] Often people think there are about five reasons to have sex, including pleasure, love, boredom, stress reduction, and procreation. When I ask this question to an auditorium of college students, and ask them to guess how many reasons there are for sex, the largest guess I've heard is fifty. However, the participants in this research study indicated 237 reasons why they have sex! The researchers grouped these reasons into four themes: physical, emotional, insecurity, and goal attainment. Some of the more shocking reasons included getting revenge, to pass on an STD/STI, to get a promotion, to make someone jealous, to feel powerful, and to have the other person stop bothering them for sex. I think this is helpful research because it leads to the realization that whatever *your* motivation is for sex, the person you're with may have very different reasons.

How might this be relevant to you? When working with couples who are facing struggles in their sex life, I like to

---

87   Cindy M. Meston and David Michael Buss, "Why Humans Have Sex," *Archives of Sexual Behavior* 36, no. 4 (2007): 477–507.

ask: "What does sex mean to you?" This question quickly gets to the heart of their different motivations for sex and often to why they're having sexual concerns. For example, when asked this question, one couple in their late thirties uncovered a host of differences. The husband liked sex for the physical release and fun, while the wife wanted sex as a way to feel accepted, beautiful, and emotionally close. For him it was a fun activity to do, but for her it was about validation and love. It's not surprising that in situations like this, he would want to be exploratory and always try new things, while she would want a slow, soft, and loving connection.

So what does sex mean to you? What motivates you, or has motivated you in the past, to have sex? The questions at the end of this chapter ask you to write down and reflect on this, but I'd also love for you to consider this question right now, as you read.

On the flip side, and often just as important, is the question: "What does *not* having sex mean to you?" For someone who is struggling with low desire, not having sex could mean feeling relief but also guilt and shame. For the partner with higher levels of desire, it could mean feeling rejected and undesirable, and also lonely and unloved. It's important to distinguish that this is what it *means* to each of you, not what is *actually* happening.

Since we're exploring what erotic topics mean to you personally, let's look at passion. What does passion mean to you? What does it feel like? When couples are going through the motions of having sex because they believe they should be having sex, or because one partner really wants it and the other participates as an obligation, passion is often a missing ingredient. Gone is that fiery energy of desire and excitement and getting lost in the moment. Sometimes people think that if their sexual interactions don't have the passion of early romance, there is something wrong. But as you'll read in this chapter, and as I referenced in my personal story at the beginning of this chapter, it's quite common for that fiery excitement to dissipate over time. You may need to expand your understanding around passion and desire, as we'll explore in a bit.

Sex matters in a lot of ways, whether you're having it regularly or not. All of the variability in quantity and quality can be fine . . . unless you're not talking about it. If you're not discussing this, you're more likely to make assumptions about what your partner is thinking or wanting. Then, in addition to your initial concerns, any differences around sexual needs can become further layered with misunderstanding and miscommunication. But just as sex can be difficult, communicating about sex can be even more difficult. Mindfulness is the perfect tool to overcome this madness, because it helps you identify your underlying emotions and motivations and how they physically impact you.

HAVING SEXUAL CONVERSATIONS

Why do so many folks struggle with talking about sex, even when they are having that conversation with someone they know, love, and trust? In the last chapter we explored the common difficulties people have with communicating everyday concerns to their partners. Now we're adding to that all the complexity that sex contributes: fears, confusion, vulnerability, defensiveness, lacking the right words, wanting to feel desirable, wanting to be seen and loved . . .

and the list goes on. In general, the reluctance to talk about sex comes down to embarrassment around sexual topics or a fear of judgment or rejection. These uncomfortable emotions can be present in everyday conversations, but sexual conversations add a new level of discomfort. Most simply, most of us were not raised with role models for good sexual communication, or even the concept that in-depth conversation about sex is important, necessary, and responsible. Most Americans go into these conversations with few skills and a lot of awkwardness. No wonder you may be avoiding these talks!

In the section Taking Responsibility for Your Triggers and Needs in chapter 3, I discussed the book *The 5 Love Languages* and the importance of owning how you most feel loved while also knowing how to fill your partner's love tank. If physical touch is your partner's love language, and sexual interactions are an important component of that, then think about how conversations about sex can be valuable to your partner. I know this might sound counterintuitive, since talking is very different from touching. However, consider this example from a heterosexual couple who had been married for almost twenty-five years and had raised one son who was out of the home. Physical touch was one of the male partner's primary love languages, but it was a pretty low priority for her. When they came to see me, they hadn't had any kind of sexual interaction in more than three years and didn't have much physical touching at all. Despite having good quality time together and a long relationship based on respect, he felt sad and rejected.

I suggested they start having weekly sensuality evenings (which I'll talk more about in the section Thinking Outside the Sexual Box later in this chapter). The intent of these evenings was to schedule time to physically connect with each other through massage, cuddling, or naked hot tub time. His love tank started getting filled, and even more so when she was enjoying the experience and connection as well.

However, after a few months of this promising progress, the couple stopped prioritizing these evenings. He was afraid she didn't really want to do them anymore, and she was avoiding bringing up the topic because she assumed that would make things worse. There's an interesting thing around love languages, though. If you ignore the topic, then not only is your partner not feeling loved, they also assume it's not even on your mind. Believing that your partner doesn't care is doubly painful. However, you can address the topic and let your partner know that you're thinking about how they want to be loved, that it matters to you, and that you'd like to get it in the calendar. This conversation indicating your concern about their physical needs goes a long way toward filling your partner's love tank—and you haven't even touched them! It's super important to follow through with your commitments, but please know that continually sharing that it's on your mind matters a lot as well.

Stating Your Sexual Needs

I get this question a lot: *How do I ask my partner to do something different sexually without hurting their feelings or making them feel overwhelmed?* We're not used to talking about sexual topics, and many of us (especially men who are socialized into traditional masculinity, but increasingly all folks nowadays) are taught that it's important to know what we're doing sexually and to be doing things "right." Therefore, it's not unusual for a partner to get defensive when you want to change something.

The first thing that can help is to facilitate a context so that your partner doesn't feel overwhelmed in the conversation. Setting a short time limit, such as twenty minutes, can be helpful in this way. Ask your partner for twenty minutes of their time to bring up a topic that matters to you. When it feels like an uncomfortable discussion could go on for a long time, your partner may be more likely to resist and shut down. But asking for a defined and limited amount of time may make them feel emotionally safer and more present. Once the twenty minutes is up, honor the time commitment, and if you have more to discuss, ask to continue at another time. If it is uncomfortable for you to drop the topic after twenty minutes, this is a good time to use the Triangle of Awareness from chapter 2 and to journal about the discomfort you're feeling.

I discussed the importance of expressing gratitude and appreciation to your partner in the previous chapter. This is also so helpful when you want to discuss sexual topics. The more your partner feels appreciated by you, and the more they know the ways in which they're already making you happy sexually, the more open they will be to hearing about what could make you even happier. It's important that you exude this appreciative and loving energy, born from a belief that your partner is already great in a lot of ways. You just know your sexual relationship could be even stronger. Otherwise, if they feel like they are failing you sexually, it's unlikely they will be able to stay open-minded and open-hearted enough to hear your request. Imagine if your partner approached you with negativity and made you feel inadequate about your sexual skills.

Would you want to listen to their needs, or would you want to defend yourself and end the conversation? Your approach with genuine caring and gratitude is important.

Next, I always tell my audiences at workshops, lectures, or online to blame it on me! Say that you read a blog, watched a video, or heard a suggestion at the talk you just attended, and that it got you thinking. Basically, you're saying that you're already happy sexually, but you've realized that there are things you didn't know that you didn't know. You're interested in exploring them with your partner, for the benefit of both of you. For the record, I rarely advocate lying or hiding things from your partner, and that's not my intent here. I am suggesting, though, a tactful and compassionate approach, knowing that these topics are difficult for many people to discuss.

While there are many sexual needs a woman might want fulfilled, over the years, I've heard a theme that surprised me—that women want to feel cherished by their partners. This is an interesting word, because I've never heard a man say that he wanted to feel cherished (although I'm sure there are some who would say that, and some women who hate this idea). As much as the feminist in me wants to dismiss this as old-fashioned, I think there is something to this idea. Naomi Wolf, in her book *Vagina*, speaks about women as Goddesses. This may feel a bit woo-woo to some readers, but there is power in what she has to say: ". . . it is obvious from putting the recent science of female sexual response side by side with Tantra 101 that when heterosexual men treat women like Goddesses—overtly—in various ways, even very everyday and manageable ways, simply verbalizing their admiration, telling them how uniquely precious they are, how beautiful they are—'the most beautiful, in their eyes'—or making gestures that show that they cherish them, this helps open up even tired, depressed, and hurt women." To Wolf, the term "Goddess" refers to a powerful woman who knows her value and knows that she deserves to get attention and be revered. She owns her alluring nature and the pleasure that she deserves.[88]

My intent is not to encourage you to be thoroughly selfish and self-absorbed, or even to take on the role of a Goddess. I mention this concept in this section on having sexual conversations because, in order to make detailed requests about your sexual needs, you need to know that your pleasure matters and that your partner cares about your pleasure. And feeling cherished and adored, whatever that means to you, may be on your list of needs. You might not have known it was on your list until you read this just now. I don't know how much of this desire comes from being raised with Disney movies with princesses, or romantic comedies in Hollywood, but I do like the nurturing and self-worth aspects of it. Whatever its origin, this is a factor that might light you up. When you're in a long-term relationship in particular, it's important to know what your partner can do to still light your inner fire after many years.

The tough thing with this need, and many other needs, is knowing how to articulate it in a way that makes sense to your partner. Unless your need is as specific as, "Please stroke my clit from top to bottom 150 times until orgasm," your requests are probably a lot more abstract

---

88   Naomi Wolf, *Vagina: A New Biography* (London: Virago, 2013), 313–314.

and ambiguous. I suggest that you do a little journaling ahead of time on the needs you'd like to state, then answer these three questions about each need:

- ▸ Why does this matter to me?
- ▸ What emotions am I hoping to feel, or what do I want to experience when this need is fulfilled?
- ▸ What are three specific, concrete things my partner can do to help me feel that way?

For example, I worked with a couple in their late twenties who had a baby boy. The wife said she wanted her husband to be more confident and in charge sexually. He wasn't sure how to do that because what brought her pleasure seemed to change from week to week, so he did regular verbal check-ins during sex. I asked her these three questions to identify the needs beneath her request, and helped translate her answers to her husband. She wanted to feel desired by her husband. She wanted to feel caught up in the moment and carried away by his passion for her. She also wanted to feel a strong, masculine energy, so that she could get out of her head and her thoughts, and just feel taken. It mattered to her because they had been together for a while, and passion didn't necessarily come easily to her anymore. As a woman in an always-aging body, she wanted to feel her husband's continuing desire for her and to feel beautiful and special.

It was hard for her to identify specific actions for him to take, so I facilitated the discussion to find concrete actions to address her request. We settled on him creating a more sensual mood in the bedroom by getting candles and scarves to hang over the lamps, thereby demonstrating that he cared about her feeling sensual and sexy in their home. We talked about how to cultivate and express confidence, what that felt like in his body, and how important it was for him to take the leap of faith that he did know how to please his wife. Then I suggested a few ways to make her feel desired, such as whispering about how her body aroused him, or telling her what he specifically wanted to do with her sexually. As they put these new ideas into action, he gained confidence stepping into a dominant role and embodying the energy of strength she wanted, and she was able to relax into her body and feel how turned on she got by feeling desired by him.

Plan Ahead and Voice Expectations

You may have experienced times when you had a specific expectation around having sex (or an expectation not to have sex), and your partner carried a different expectation in their head. Neither of you spoke about it ahead of time, so you both assumed that your partner shared your expectations. I worked with one couple who enjoyed their quality time when they visited their mountain vacation home together. Inevitably, though, he would become distant and irritable because they weren't having more sex. He, like many higher-desire partners, had a specific expectation of frequent sex while on vacation, in particular when they woke up in the morning. She was not opposed to this idea overall and enjoyed their sexual interactions, but sleeping in later was an important part of vacation enjoyment for her. So when he woke up and wanted sex, and she asked for more sleep, he became sullen and felt rejected. She, on the other hand, was irritated and had trouble falling back asleep. However, once we talked through the specifics of what each expected and hoped for, and found a balance to meet both of their needs (he would walk the dog and work out while she continued to sleep, and then shower and rejoin her in bed), they were able to avoid this common vacation miscommunication.

While vacations are the main context for assumptions around sexual frequency that have surfaced in my private practice, holidays and weekends can also create expectations. It seems that any time your schedule is out of the ordinary in some way, there may be expectations of more or less sex. If this has been problematic in your relationship before, the most straightforward way to avoid this is to sit down and have a talk ahead of time. Gently point out that you know there have been hurt feelings in the past because of unstated expectations, so you want to clear the air about what both of you are thinking. This proactive approach to addressing expectations is a great practice to add to your sexual communication repertoire.

Sexual Consent

Consent is a hot topic right now, especially on college campuses, partly because of the #MeToo movement. But consent is relevant at all times in all sexual interactions. Consent refers to all parties being open to and interested in the physical and sexual activities they are participating in, without feeling forced, pressured, or coerced. It's my belief that anyone who was trained in traditional masculine values in the United States learned that they were supposed to push to get what they want sexually. They aren't taught that this is disrespectful or problematic, but rather that this is how they show strength and get what they want. They are often taught that the other person actually wants the same thing that they do, so verbal consent is unnecessary. And they are also taught that women are just being coy or trying to protect their reputations as "good girls" by saying no when they really mean yes.

If you grew up being trained in traditional feminine characteristics, you learned to be passive, quieter, and caring towards others. In a sexual situation, you learned to be responsible, but you were also taught to be nice and to defer to the needs of others. Although you were supposed to look pretty, you were not taught that *your* sexual pleasure should ever be a priority. This training clearly impacts women's sexual decision making and sexual experiences. Those of us who have received this training often don't even realize that there could be another way.

I shared a personal story of a sexual boundary violation at a storytelling event in May 2016, called "Sex & the Price of Masculinity"; the video was released a couple of months later on YouTube.[89] It was an uncomfortably vulnerable story to share in a public way, but I knew that sexual coercion happens much too often. I figured that if I shared my story, I could also bring my sociological and sexological background into explaining why I thought it happened and how we can create a new narrative around sexual consent communication. I believe that sexual coercion, from mild to blunt, is built into the fabric of traditional masculine and feminine roles in the United States.

A lot of folks present sexual consent as a straightforward topic, and it should be. But, as with any commu-

---

89   You can watch the video here: youtu.be/MOSU7B8iR-Q

nication, it's often open to misinterpretation in practice. I think this is part of the reason we're so bad at this as a society. There are so many assumptions around sexual interactions, but we don't seem to *realize* that we're making assumptions. I often use the example of going out to dinner with someone and allowing them to order from the menu, based on their tastes, mood, or desires. You don't just assume that you know what that person wants to eat, when, and how much. And you certainly don't just shove food into their mouth. You let them use their voice and have a choice. Yet somehow, something as personal and individualized as sexuality is not seen as worthy of the same respect. I chalk a lot of this up to the insufficient sex education offered in our country and our shame-based approach to bodies and sex. We just don't talk about it enough in a responsible and educational way. Nor do we help folks gain skills in working through the emotional and social awkwardness. It would be beneficial to all if we could create new social norms around sex that grasp its complexity.

Consent is also nuanced because we sometimes feel conflicted about whether to engage in sexual interactions. For example, women have been trained to be nice and not rock the boat, as I discussed in detail in chapter 1. This might mean that you're not really interested in doing a specific sexual activity, but you don't stop it because doing so would feel incredibly awkward and inappropriate (like the client story I shared at the start of chapter 1). You *want* the other person to like you, to be attracted to you. So halting a sexual act that another person assumes is the next step can feel very uncomfortable. This is why I teach mindfulness to help us all find our voice sexually. The more we are aware of the madness—our belief systems and emotions, and where they live in us—the more we can make new choices that are aligned with our values. When you've trained yourself to sit with your fears and demons, you're not as afraid to face them in a sexual situation.

The other side of healthy consent conversations involves being able to handle rejection. Rejection feels personal and raw. But the experience of rejection includes a lot of interpretation (think the Thoughts part of the Triangle), which means that the situation is open to more empowering interpretations. I'm part of a fantastic group called Sex Positive San Diego. We create educational and experiential spaces for people to learn about everything from sexual shame to polyamory, kink, pleasure, and societal values. In these spaces, people can experience shame- and judgment-free environments to explore new aspects of their sexual and sensual pleasure. One of the things I love the most about this group is how we teach consent. To address the very real, uncomfortable feelings of rejection, we teach how to appreciate a "no." For example, if you ask (in an appropriate sexual context) to touch another person's nipples and they say no, you could sulk, get angry, or take it personally, OR you could say, "Thank you for taking care of yourself." Seriously. You don't know why the other person is saying no, but you do know that they said no because it wasn't something they wanted right now. Which means they were taking care of themselves and their needs.[90]

However, it can be a challenge to switch to this mode

---

[90]   Thank you to Sex Positive Los Angeles and Sex Positive San Diego for teaching this to me, and to sex educator Reid Mihalko for creating this sexual consent template.

of thinking, as it requires quite a bit of mindfulness. You have to first notice the uncomfortable negative raw feeling, which may be accompanied by the belief that you're unwanted. Then you must accept that discomfort in the moment without blaming the other person or emotionally withdrawing. Finally, you have to make the genuine choice to be kind to the person in front of you. If you choose this path of kindness to yourself and your partners, it is a revolutionary way to turn rejection into appreciation.

BLOCKS TO DESIRE

You are normal. I'm going to say that again. *You are normal.* There is such a large range of sexual desires, appetites, body shapes and sizes (including genitals and breasts), and erotic thoughts. As long as your sexual activities are consensual and legal, they are normal and fine. I hate the word "normal," actually, because it implies a black-and-white view of what's okay and what's not regarding sexuality. But I use this term here because that is the term that many people use, and if they're not speaking about it, they're thinking and worrying about it.

Several factors play into how we experience desire and whether we want to act on that desire. There is a physiological component, which is what we often call "feeling horny." This is that yearning and pull towards a sexual encounter or a sexual release. Our emotional and mental states, and how they interact, are another factor. Do you feel appreciated by your partner, or stressed, or frustrated and disappointed? Our wide range of emotions and thoughts (imagine the Triangle here, and all those thoughts, emotions, and bodily sensations that we have throughout any day) play a large role in our interest in sexual activities. The final piece is our values and beliefs. These are the factors I addressed in chapter 1, including all the madness of our cultural learnings. Do you think your body fits the approved standards of beauty? Are there certain sexual acts that you deem morally unacceptable? Your physiological, emotional, and mental states mix together with your cultural learnings to impact your sexual desire.

When it comes to specific blocks to your desire, there can be many. These obstacles put the "brakes" on your sexual desire. In the fantastic book *Come as You Are: The Surprising New Science That Will Transform Your Sex Life*, author Emily Nagoski writes about the dual control model of sexual response, which states that we all have two "pedals" controlling our sexual desire and arousal: an accelerator and a brake. Clearly we're talking about the brakes here—the factors that inhibit feeling turned on sexually.[91] But later in this chapter, particularly in the Thinking Outside the Sexual Box section, I'll address how to press your sexual accelerator pedal!

Some of the blocks to feeling desire, such as harmful messages you learned growing up, a negative body image, not feeling loved and nurtured in the way that's meaningful to you, being in your head instead of being present in your body, improper handling of resentments, and unfavorable timing and availability, have been or will be addressed in other sections of this book. So this section delves into a few other specific blocks and how you can

---

91   Emily Nagoski, *Come as You Are: The Surprising New Science That Will Transform Your Sex Life* (New York: Simon & Schuster, 2015).

use mindful awareness to make a shift. The reason I go into such detail about blocks to desire is because, as one female client shared, "It's very empowering to be able to identify what it is so you can work on removing it. It gives you power over how you feel."

Overwhelmed with Discomfort

There is one block to sexual desire that is foundational to all the other blocks: the impulse to run away from discomfort. But discomfort can only be addressed and worked through by choosing to stay present with it. My suggestion here is to use the basic mindfulness skills we've already discussed, but with a slight twist. For example, notice when you have some sort of fear, disgust, dislike, or angst around the thought of being sexual with your partner. Perhaps focus on that thought and those sensations right now, if this resonates with you. Then, instead of identifying your thoughts, emotions, and bodily sensations, notice *just* your bodily sensations. As the Buddhist nun Pema Chödrön said, "Drop the story and stay with your feelings."[92] What she means is to allow the story you're telling yourself, and the meaning and values you attach to it, to slip away. Then choose to drop into your body and raw sensations. You might be thinking, *I love my partner, so there must be something wrong with me that I don't want to have sex. I should just do it anyway.* If you drop this story and pay attention *only* to the sensations in your body, you might notice that your heart is beating faster, your hands are clenched,

---

92   Pema Chödrön, *Getting Unstuck: Breaking Your Habitual Patterns and Encountering Naked Reality* (Boulder, Colo.: Sounds True, 2005). Audiobook.

and there's a prickly feeling below your chest and a hollowed sensation in your gut. *That* is what's real in that moment.

It can be scary to stay present with such raw sensations, so perhaps choose to close your eyes and do it for only a few seconds at a time before opening your eyes. But then close your eyes again and dive back into your sensations. If you notice that you're still distracted by the story, perhaps this time with thoughts like *My partner hasn't even tried to fill my love tank and doesn't care, so why should I want to have sex anyway?*, just shift your focus onto your bodily sensations each time you notice the distraction. The more you practice this, the longer you can stay present with such discomfort. You can do this "noticing" exercise anytime a block to sexual activity arises, or as a short, planned activity prior to engaging in sexual activity. Don't forget to be compassionate with yourself through the process and honor that you are experiencing emotional pain.

Continue to identify *where* you feel the discomfort in your body. Is it in your chest? Throat? Solar plexus? Gut? There is no specific end goal for this process or set amount of time to do it. But if you fully feel these sensations and accept them in the moment (recall that the second A of the Three A's of mindfulness is Acceptance), they will often dissipate in just a couple minutes. If it's helpful, remind yourself that these are just feelings in your body, that they will pass, and that they don't have to control you. Remember that your discomfort here likely stems from the madness you've inherited from our society. Your body is doing what it is trained to do, which is to warn you with uncomfortable sensations when you feel socially threatened. Through mindfulness, though, you don't have to get stuck here anymore.

As odd as it might sound, feeling like you need to have sex when you don't want to, even with a loving partner, *is* socially threatening. We are innately social creatures as humans, so we're wired to have strong fears around losing our social connections. However, you probably recognize at this point that running from discomfort isn't working to protect you, because it causes you to avoid important topics or close your heart to an intimate connection. You can start to make the choice that you no longer want this protection to block you or shut down your heart. Making that choice is the first step in learning how to breathe through and stay present with your discomfort, and therefore be able to gently expand your comfort zone around sexual conversations, topics, and activities. Sit calmly through the discomfort, while also recognizing that this is legitimate suffering. Then continue to have compassion for your suffering, and perhaps even for all those who suffer in a similar way.[93] We are all in this emotional turmoil of life together.

Distractions or Worries

Feeling distracted is another block to desire that is directly related to mindfulness. If you are choosing to be in a sexual encounter with your partner but are having trouble getting your head into the action, notice what exactly is distracting you. Are you thinking about chores that need

---

93   I'm referencing the Buddhist practice of *tonglen*, where you choose to breathe in the suffering of others, with recognition of the common humanity of suffering, and breathe out compassion and loving-kindness for yourself and others.

to be done? Are you wondering what you're missing on your Instagram feed? Are you worried about sexually disappointing your partner? Are you having negative thoughts or worries about your body? Are you resentful that you "have to" be sexual in that moment? These all may be normal thoughts. But if you want to get turned on, they can clearly get in the way of allowing your body to sexually kick in. To choose an alternative path, I recommend a three-step process:

- ▸ Recognize and acknowledge that you are distracted, and identify what the thought is about.
- ▸ If you're distracted by negative thoughts about yourself or worries about your sexual abilities, *thank your brain* for having that thought. I know this sounds ridiculous, since they are negative thoughts, but they are only popping up because at some emotional level, they are trying to protect you from getting hurt by the person you're with. So thank your thoughts for trying to protect you, and then tell yourself: *I've got this. I'm okay.*
- ▸ Actively choose to focus your attention on one (or all five) of your senses.

You might have to do this over and over again, every time you notice yourself feeling distracted or worried. That's fine. If your distracting thoughts aren't negative, but just random thoughts popping up, you can do just the first and third steps. This is all a process, and eventually over time you will retrain your brain not to shift to worries or distractions, but to stay in the moment.

Loss of Trust

A lack of trust in your partner, as it relates to your desire or arousal, often surfaces because of infidelity. If your partner has cheated on you, it makes sense that you're reluctant to be sexual with them. All of the mindfulness activities and communication techniques in this book are helpful when you choose to stay with a partner through infidelity, because they help you stay present and responsible, despite your pain around this loss of trust. I suggest ongoing activities in your relationship that build appreciation, trust, and communication. The conflict resolution, attentive listening, and weekly acknowledgments practices in chapter 3 are helpful in this regard (all the exercises in this book are listed with their page numbers in chapter 7). They can increase your vulnerable interactions and understanding of each other, thereby rebuilding your trust. If you notice distracting thoughts about the cheating while you're sexually interacting with your partner, the same three-step process for distractions will be helpful.

Trust is a vital component of any relationship; it takes time to build, and likewise takes time to rebuild. If you're both choosing to stay together after a breach of trust like this, it is up to your partner to continue to show that they are worthy of your trust, and it's your responsibility to take that continual leap of faith every day to open your heart enough to trust again.

Many women speak about their lack of intuition regarding their partner's cheating and ask how they can learn to trust themselves again as well. Do you trust your intuition? Do you know how to access your intuition? I believe that our intuition reveals itself in layers, and the more we gain deep knowledge about ourselves, the more we can hear and understand the nuances of our inner voice. Intuition often shows up as a gut feeling and deep sense of knowing, despite no logical evidence. However, patterned behaviors based on fears and past negative experiences can also show up as a gut feeling (e.g., you don't want to be cheated on again, so now everything makes you suspicious).

I've found that my intuition is quite strong and accurate when I'm fully present in a situation, and when I'm in a state of open-heartedness or compassion. However, if I'm feeling threatened emotionally, or if one of my emotional triggers has been activated, I react from defensiveness, fear, or hurt, not from intuition. As discussed in chapter 2, daily practices of sitting quietly, with a focus on breath, the present moment, and observing thoughts and bodily sensations without judgment, further develop an important part of our prefrontal cortex that better integrates the main parts of the brain. If you need to rebuild trust in a partner and trust in yourself, starting a daily meditation practice may be in order.

Stuck in Saying No

Several years ago I took six months of improv comedy classes. It was so much harder than I thought it would be! We would play various games on stage in small groups. One of the games that was particularly hard, but fun, was called "Fresh Choice." As we created a scene together, trying to follow the rules of improv we had been taught, a "referee" could blow a whistle and demand, "Fresh choice!" after any statement we made. This meant that we would have to say something completely different from what we had just said. It's no easy task to mentally shift gears like that. But it is a helpful game to consider using when you're feeling stuck in a situation with your partner.

For example, I had a client who was a woman in her late thirties with nine-year-old twins, and every time her boyfriend expressed interest in sex, without thought, she responded "no." She started playing with a "fresh choice" mindset, which meant that when she said or thought *no*, she would mindfully catch herself and offer a different choice. Sometimes she would say *maybe*, or sometimes she would counteroffer for a later time. Other times she asked for help finishing a task or a few minutes of meaningful conversation about their day to feel more connected and potentially open to sexual connection.

Fears around expectations can also lead to continually saying no. These fears include sexual expectations that you think your partner has, the expectations you're putting on yourself to perform, or the expectations of what you think it means to be a sexual woman. These assumptions of what's expected are likely shaped by the madness messages from your youth, and may feel like impossible standards. It's helpful to get clear on your expectations, so that you can voice them to your partner to get feedback and find out if they are accurate. The expectations that we believe others have of us in life can be a heavy weight. But in the sexual realm, with someone we care about in such an intimate setting, those expectations can feel heavy enough to shut down our desire. I included a question about this in this chapter's Reflection & Writing section so that you can explore this important block with greater depth and clarity.

Don't Know Your Own Pleasure

You might have grown up learning that your sexual arousal and pleasure are the responsibility of your partner, which means another human being is expected to know your body and read your mind. Which isn't fair, and isn't ideal for you to actually experience pleasure to the depths that are possible. But if I ask you what turns you on, what feels good, and how you like to be touched, can you answer those questions? What are your specific erotic zones? How do you like to have your genitals touched and not touched? What fantasies turn you on? If you cannot answer these questions in detail, then I have two suggested activities.

The first suggestion is called Meditative Masturbation. I love this name—Meditative Masturbation—because it's two words that we never hear together. But why shouldn't we? Both activities are self-nurturing and ideally help you get to know yourself better. Meditative Masturbation is a mindful approach to masturbation: choosing to direct your focus on exploring your erotic areas with fingers and/or toys, and, when you notice distracting thoughts or self-judgment, choosing to bring your focus back to your observed sensations. Remember that a key component of mindfulness is accepting what you notice and having compassion for your experience. And you certainly deserve compassion! If you feel embarrassed about touching your-self—or if you never thought it was okay to learn about your own pleasure—then this exploration is a radical stance against your teachings of sexual madness.

This practice is meant to reduce any shame, embarrassment, or discomfort you might have around masturbating and give you permission to learn what does feel good. Just like you might have taken the time early in a relationship to set the romantic mood for a sexual encounter, you should do the same for yourself during Meditative Masturbation, in terms of ambience, music, and coziness. You could dim the lights, light a candle, or pull a warm blanket around you. Then gently explore touching your body without the endpoint of orgasm in mind. I encourage you to check out the ten-minute guided audio file on Meditative Masturbation that you can listen to for free on my website, which leads you through such a sensual exploration: www.drjennsden.com/meditative -masturbation/

My second suggested activity is to write down five peak sexual experiences you've had. By peak sexual experiences, I mean sexual encounters you've had in the past that stand out as the most erotic, hot, passionate, exciting, or romantic. Whether with your current partner, a past partner, or even on your own, write down what stands out in your memory—moments that probably even make you feel a little randy just thinking about them right now. You can also include sexual fantasies that you have when masturbating, or something that you read in erotica or saw in porn. Basically, you're looking for what has made you feel really hot, even if you're embarrassed by it. Spend some time writing down these experiences and exploring what surfaces for you. Remember not to judge yourself on what turns you on.

These exploratory activities will provide you with important information about what's already wired into

your brain for sexual arousal. Once you have this information, consider what pieces of this you might be able
to bring into your current sex life—an activity, position,
place, style, energy, or dialogue. On the other hand, if
one of your peak sexual memories or fantasies is something that you would never actually want to do in your
current situation, something that's totally normal as a
fantasy but could be dangerous in real life (e.g., sex with
a stranger on a train), consider whether you could have
your partner whisper some of that fantasy to you while
you're together. Also consider what "feel" you are trying
to create, in terms of the energy you want your partner to
bring to the situation (e.g., dominant, aggressive, obse-
quious, reprimanding, confident, loving, warm). Explain
this to your partner in as much detail as you can and ask
that they be incredibly compassionate and nonjudgmental
with this vulnerable information you're sharing. Then
slowly start working together to bring that energy to your
sexual interactions.

Stress and Children

Not surprisingly, stress, and its mental and physical rami-
fications, can directly impact our sexual health. When
we're stressed and feeling overburdened, we're more likely
to focus on negative events in the past or pessimistic
expectations of the future, rather than being present in our
bodies in any given moment. Stress is wanting something
to be different from the way it is. Wanting traffic to clear
up. Wanting more time to complete something. Wishing
your kids weren't talking back to you. We can feel powerless, overwhelmed, and tired, which is pretty much the
opposite of sexy and sexual. Also, stress has been found

to have a negative impact on our sex hormones, leaving us with a lower libido. (Unless you're part of the 10 to 20 percent of the population who are more sexually interested when they are stressed, according to Emily Nagoski![94])

Remember the mindfulness exercises I wrote about in chapter 2—the ones about becoming present to your five senses, at a stoplight or at home, and the doorway breathing reminder? These are great tools to integrate into your day for stress reduction. Every time you're at a stoplight, focus on one of your senses and notice what arises while taking deep breaths. Every time you walk through a doorway, use it as a signal to take even just one deep breath as a reminder that you don't have to feel stress in that moment. Or download the mindfulness bell app I mentioned in that chapter and set it to ring at random times during the day. When it chimes, take a few deep breaths and anchor yourself in the moment with your five senses. With practice and repetition, you can retrain your brain to be less reactive to stress.

All of these stresses and remedies relate to raising children as well. Although they are the joys of your life, children also take a lot of your time and emotional energy and challenge your willpower. This can make it hard to want to give more of *you* to your partner in a sexual way. Many new moms feel (rightfully so) that their bodies are not their own anymore, but that they belong to their babies. On top of that, societal messages put great emphasis on being a "supermom" and tackling all of life with graceful perfection—an impossible and unfair pressure to place on any mother.

---

94   Nagoski, *Come as You Are*, 118.

I spoke to a new mother once, a woman in her late twenties, who felt so physically spent at the end of the day, between breastfeeding and caring for her eight-month-old, that she actually recoiled in disgust at her husband's touch. Clearly this was a dangerous precedent to set moving forward, and it needed to be nipped in the bud before it did serious damage to both of them. Ultimately, she needed to feel that she and her husband were more of a team; that the weight and stress of the new baby wasn't all on her shoulders. She also wanted him to approach her body in a nonsexual way first, without an energy of expectation, because his approach had started to feel predatory. When he focused on approaching her with the intention of love and nurturing, she was able to relax and start to open up to him again.

Overall, anything that creates stress, frustration, or overwhelming feelings can be addressed in a healthy way through mindfulness and meditation. One of my clients from many years ago bought a mindfulness bell, which is a small bell that is struck with a wooden mallet, for her living room. She wanted to use it with her children when they were out of control, to remind everyone to pause and take several deep breaths. The funny thing was, her nine-year-old daughter started using it every time she discerned her mom was stressed. At first my client was irritated by this, but over time she came to see it as a gift and to realize that even her daughter was her teacher. There is much research showing the stress-reducing capacity of regular mindfulness and meditation practices. If you find yourself chronically stressed, I highly recommend a regular practice.

Fertility Concerns

Wanting a baby with your partner is a beautiful thing. But trying for a long time to no avail, whether on your own or with medical intervention, can create tension and hurt feelings. The pressure of being sexual at an appointed time and the continual disappointment each month when you're not pregnant can be devastating to an otherwise connected, loving partnership. If you're taking additional hormones, that can wreak havoc with your emotions and mental states. You may blame yourself or your partner, or shut your heart down from the pain. Mindfulness can be incredibly helpful in maintaining or repairing your relationship.

Regarding the pressure around scheduled sex, I suggest saying the following affirmation aloud when you're about to have sex: "We cannot control whether or not this leads to pregnancy. But we can control how we interact with each other and how we care for each other. So let's just love each other." Feel free to play with it and make it your own. Look into each other's eyes, take a few breaths together, and genuinely contemplate the love that you have for each other that brought you to this bedroom in the first place. Intentionally focus on opening your heart center. This would also be a good time to throw in a few statements of gratitude for each other, to focus on what is good and strong already. Feel the opening, warmth, and expansion in your heart center during these interactions. And if saying something like this feels cheesy and makes you both laugh, that's perfect, because that laughter can ease the pressure and tension.

With all the mindfulness and communication tools I've discussed already, you have a lot at your fingertips to make sure you're both creating a safe space to discuss the difficulty and disappointment of your fertility process. Be a team with each other. Let this distressing process bring you closer together through compassion, instead of serving as a disconnecting wedge. This is hard, but you can do hard. Be compassionate to your partner and also remember every day to do something that is mindfully nurturing for yourself.

Sexual Abuse

You may have experienced sexual trauma in your past. First off, I'm sorry that you've had to deal with such a difficult and unfair experience. You're in good company with many strong women around the world who are survivors. Your experience probably had an impact on your sexuality in one way or another, although this does not mean that you're broken. It just means that someone has been unkind to you, and your mind and body have done the best they could from then on to try to protect you from being hurt again. It can also mean that there is some sexual confusion that got wired into your brain in terms of who you can trust and how to trust, and how to put up healthy boundaries. Not surprisingly, mindfulness is a powerful tool to learn who you are as a sexual woman on your own terms, and how to stand in that power and knowledge in a responsible yet kind way.

It is beyond the scope of this book to address the topics of sexual abuse and assault with the depth they deserve; processing these negative experiences is best done with a counselor or therapist specializing in these areas. I do want to offer, however, a simple suggestion if you feel you're in a good place to take this on. First, remind yourself that what happened is in the past, and although it still lives in you, in *this* actual moment, as you read this book, you're okay. Anchor yourself to this moment with your five senses and observe the safety and stability in what's happening right now.

I had a client who was afraid of being sexual with her boyfriend because she didn't want to have a flashback to when she was sexually abused as a child by a relative. She was concerned that she would start connecting her boyfriend to those negative memories. Her fears of this happening would often surface during the day when she was at work. When she started doing the five senses observation (see page 92), though, and shifted from being stuck in old thought patterns to being in her body in the present day, her fear would abate. Once she had done this a few times, she began to realize that she had more control than she thought, and she started feeling empowered in the moment, instead of fearful and powerless. She also took this exercise into the bedroom with her, and, when any fears or memories arose, she would touch the sheets, listen to the music, smell her partner, and remind herself that *in this moment* she was in control and safe.

Side Effects of Medications

This is a tough one. Whether you're taking birth control because you want to avoid pregnancy, or you're on antidepressants because of their value in maintaining your emotional and mental balance, medications can impact your sexual functioning. It's not uncommon to experience lowered desire, a reduced ability to get aroused, or difficulty having an orgasm as side effects from some of these medications. This puts you in a quandary, because the medication is serving a valuable function for your happiness. Although it can be embarrassing, this is a significant topic to discuss with your health care practitioner so they know that the sexual side effects are impacting your quality of life. You may then be able to try a new medication that won't decrease your desire or sexual functioning in the same way.

If you don't have a choice about which medication you're taking, it's important to first acknowledge the change in your sexuality and discuss it openly with your partner. Then, as a couple, you can work to accept this as your new normal. However, I want to remind you that acceptance does not mean complacency. After acceptance, the next step is to think outside the box about your sexual activities and be open to trying new ideas. The section Thinking Outside the Sexual Box later in this chapter is all about this approach.

GIVING YOURSELF PERMISSION

You may wonder why I have a section about permission, and what permission has to do with mindfulness in the realm of sex, passion, and desire. But ask yourself the following questions: Do you give yourself permission to be sexy? Permission to be sexual? Permission to follow your passion? Permission to be sexual on your own terms? Permission to say yes? Permission to say no? Permission to be happy? Permission to take care of your body, nurture your emotions, and slow down when you need to? It seems funny that we even have to think this way, but as women we're often taught to place the needs of others first and to always give unconditionally of ourselves. If we don't consciously choose to give ourselves permission for self-care—physically, mentally, emotionally, socially, and spiritually—it might not happen.

I spoke to a group of sixty female dentists about this topic, and afterwards, one of the women came up to me. She said, "I wish I had heard this message thirty years ago so I would have realized that I didn't have to be everything to everyone and run myself into the ground." For many women, it doesn't occur to them that they could behave any other way.

This struggle with giving yourself permission can be connected to other obstacles that we've discussed in this chapter. In order to give yourself permission, you must first understand your own needs. You also have to understand that you're worthy of having those needs fulfilled. So many women are undermined and sucked into a belief system that keeps them in a constant emotional battle with their bodies and sexuality. This often means that they carry a lot of shame, and to reiterate Brené Brown's words "Shame is the intensely painful feeling or experience of believing that we are flawed and therefore unworthy of love and belonging."[95] It's important to know your value as a woman, and as a sexual woman, even though you may feel imperfect. We are all imperfect, and there truly is no version of being "perfect sexually" or "perfectly sexual." Often when we look at what gets in the way of our goals or personal growth, we look to external factors and other people, not realizing the power we have to grant ourselves permission.

When you're creating new personal belief systems, I like to suggest the use of mantras. My version of a mantra is a phrase that you can repeat when you've been triggered and

---

95   Brown, *The Gifts of Imperfection*, 39.

sent into an old pattern. It reminds you of your strengths, or that you are committed to a healthier path. A mantra can help snap you out of your habit, and sometimes that's enough of a change to refocus your attention. A powerful one that I've used in various forms with clients is this: "I give myself permission to be on the journey (or path) of being an empowered sexual woman." You're not saying you *are* an empowered sexual woman or have reached any specific goal, so you're less likely to evoke mental resistance. This just simply gives you permission to be on an exploratory journey with a general goal. For someone struggling with self-worth, an appropriate mantra could be: "I am on the journey to knowing I'm good enough." If this resonates with you, try it out right now!

Some women learn that their sexual identity—who they are as a sexual being—is defined by the partner they're with. If you identify as heterosexual, then you might have been exposed to the belief that sexual activity is male terrain, and it's a woman's responsibility to follow his lead. I've had female clients in their fifties who were recently divorced, who didn't know who they were sexually without the partner they had been with for thirty years. So an important part of giving yourself sexual permission is to give yourself permission to define what and how you want to be sexual, even if you're slowly learning what this means.

As you're working your way through this topic, check in and see if you notice any shame arising. Brené Brown writes, "Shame is that warm feeling that washes over us, making us feel small, flawed, and never good enough."[96]

---

96   Brown, *The Gifts of Imperfection*, 38.

Think about this visceral description, with its accompanying beliefs, as you read the rest of this section. If you notice that you think you can't do the exercises or make these shifts in beliefs, or don't want to read further, that might be a sign that the text has triggered a shame response. That's okay. Just use your new mindfulness skills to notice where the feelings are located, have compassion for yourself for these difficult feelings, and then take some deep breaths and allow this emotional reaction to pass on its own.

Playing with Neutral

What if you decided to momentarily discard what you "know" you like and dislike regarding sexual activity? By this, I mean that you go into a sexual encounter without any preconceived notions about what you like or don't like, and just stay open. Try this on for a moment. Presuming you are in a loving context with someone you trust, what if you decided to be "neutral" about sexual activities? I know this is actually impossible to do, and you can't forget what you already know, but I'm suggesting a shift in the energy that you bring to sexual interactions.

For example, say you "know" that you hate giving blowjobs. They are tiring, not arousing, taste bad, feel demeaning, or whatever meaning you've attached to that experience. But what if you decided to play with feeling neutral about going down on a male partner? Perhaps approach the activity as a learning experience, as a way to listen to the nuances of your partner's responses, or to find new details about the penis and balls in front of you. Consider also what could potentially make the experience more pleasurable for you, such as being touched at the same time, hearing words of affirmation while you give it, showering together beforehand, or using a tasty lubricant. In the long run, giving a blowjob still might not be at the top of your favorite sex activities, and that's totally fine. But you've given yourself a chance to reclaim this activity in a potentially empowering or appreciative way. By playing with neutral, you now have a new choice about how you feel about that activity. As referenced earlier, our preferences and comforts keep us in a cage. Switching to a neutral mindset can break down those walls.

Permission to "Disappoint" Your Partner

I was working with a heterosexual couple who had been married for six years and had a ten-year-old daughter, and although we were making some progress in their sexual connection, the wife (who was in her mid-thirties) wasn't doing my suggested homework and avoided detailed conversations about it. She didn't have much interest in sex, and said she rarely did unless she was drinking alcohol. But her healthy diet and lifestyle were at odds with that. She didn't even want to flirt with her husband, because that felt inappropriate to her. In an individual session, we uncovered a goldmine of relevant information about her youth and some sketchy experiences she had had with trusted males. As soon as she was deemed sexually attractive in adolescence by her male friends, she was the target of unwanted attention and uncomfortable comments. Over the years, being overtly sexual, flirty, or even perceived as sexy had felt dangerous and unsafe.

This was a smart defensive mechanism she had unwittingly put into place, but at this point in her life, it was getting in the way of intimacy with her husband. I asked her to visualize what it would feel like just to flirt with her husband, with no expectation of sex. Then, through the Triangle of Awareness, we identified the following information: She believed it was inappropriate to flirt because he would have expectations; she was afraid of disappointing him; she felt fear and anxiety about bringing that kind of attention to herself; and she viscerally felt the fear in her chest and up into her throat. As she identified all of these details, and she sat with me discussing these uncomfortable emotions, I pointed out that she had the strength to face them. She didn't have to avoid these uncomfortable feelings anymore.

My client realized that her past defenses were blocking her from expressing her sexuality. We talked through some simple ways to start flirting (e.g., texts during the day, a slap on the ass in the kitchen, or a whisper when out with friends about how she might want him to touch her later). She felt more equipped to commit to these fun interactions with her husband and move through her fears. I also made sure that *he* knew to accept these flirtations without expectations for sex, and that this was meant to bring a flirtier and lighter energy overall to their relationship.

You have permission to just flirt. You also have permission to meet only a small percentage of the physical pleasure you believe your partner desires. Many women presume their partner wants and needs sex to be the most passionate and amazing experience each time. But when I've asked the partner with higher desire, they admit that it would be great, but it's not necessary. They realize that it's not realistic to have that level of sexual ecstasy every time. I suggested to one late-twenties client to shoot for meeting only thirty percent of the sexual pleasure she believed her husband wanted. She had enjoyed their sexual encounters early in the marriage and wanted to return to that, but resentments and fears had grown so big that she just avoided physical closeness. I encouraged her to use the mantra: "Whatever I bring is enough. I am enough." Lowering her self-expectations, and being kind to herself, removed the pressure to be "sexually perfect" and allowed her just to show up and enjoy some physical pleasure with her husband. This shift in her expectations meant she gave herself permission to be sexual again, at whatever level she could.

Permission to be a "Naughty Girl"

If you grew up with the "good girl" mentality like many of us do in the United States, being a "naughty girl" may feel foreign to you. You might judge "naughty girls" harshly because of their openness to pursuing sexual pleasure. You also might secretly want to be more of a "naughty girl," wishing to feel freer and more desired by your partner for being sexually open. When it comes down to it, there is nothing particularly "good" about being a "good girl," and nothing "naughty" about being a "naughty girl." They are just sexual labels we learn growing up. That being said, giving yourself permission to be freer with sexual words and actions *is* a good thing.

Dirty talk during sexual play can be a way of channeling your inner naughty girl. Part of taking this on is becoming comfortable with sexual terminology and with using your voice during sexual interactions. If you're new to dirty talk, your discomfort could range from feeling awkward to feeling out-and-out ridiculous. And that's all okay. Like any new skill, there is a learning curve, and it's not uncommon to feel silly along the way. There is a strong "fake it until you make it" component to gaining comfort with dirty talk. I recommend finding some erotica you like and reading it aloud to yourself to build your tolerance with the discomfort. It might take a bit of research to find erotica that turns you on, which is why I recommend short stories to efficiently sample a lot of styles. Hearing your own voice speak sexual words will start to normalize them, as well as give you ideas for the kinds of things you might like saying (or doing).

I had a female client who was visibly uncomfortable with what she called "raunchy" talk. Through discussion, we realized she was grouping all spoken sexual words under one umbrella of inappropriate and uncomfortable language. I helped her differentiate between "raunchy" talk and "raw" talk—talk that was about what she wanted and what her husband was doing, but that didn't feel debasing to her. We all have our own lines we can draw regarding what words to use, but I do encourage you to question why you don't like certain terminology and mindfully reflect on that. Overall, this process can be particularly valuable to overcome sexual embarrassment and shame.

Owning Your Desire

By "owning" your desire, I mean taking responsibility for it. We generally think that desire is something that happens *to us* or something that our partner is responsible for evoking. But only you can know when you feel desire and what specifically arouses you at any given moment—your partner is not a mind reader. If you're struggling to feel the levels of desire you'd like to with your partner,

I suggest you take on some personal exploration to find what does turn you on. Find where your erotic energy lives in your body and how you can choose to awaken that. This is a process of mindful discovery around the nuances of your sexual desire.

The first step is to pay attention to times when you do feel horny already. If your body isn't naturally and frequently asking for sex, pay attention to any times when you do feel more sexual or open to sex. If you're not taking hormonal birth control (which stops you from ovulating) and you're not postmenopausal, you may notice a surge in physical desire for sexual activity around ovulation, which is roughly halfway between the start of your periods. Use this hornier time period to your advantage, and perhaps even plan ahead in your calendar. When you know you're going to be ovulating, and therefore feeling a physical yearning for intimacy, schedule a date night so you and your partner have quality time with each other. Give this desire a chance to expand and take hold, and facilitate closeness with your partner to increase the likelihood of a sexual encounter.

The second place to look is at what primes your pump physically and sexually. I hear many women say how difficult it can be to switch from their "everyday" mode of how they move through the world to their "sexual" mode. Although folks with higher levels of desire may move about their day constantly on the verge of feeling sexual, so that it doesn't take much to tip the scales, many others do not regularly embody sexual energy in that way. And when you're tired, overworked, stressed, or overwhelmed, sexual feelings can seem really distant. So taking responsibility for "priming your pump" means determining what helps you switch from everyday mode to a place where your juices start pumping.

Use the following questions to help guide this process of gliding into a sexual mode: What thoughts or actions help you to feel a bit of desire? If you fantasize about a past, really hot sexual experience, does that turn you on? Can you visualize something exciting you've seen in porn or read in erotica? Does remembering a time when you felt physically and emotionally close to your partner help you feel that way now? These kinds of questions and visualizations will hopefully shift your mind into a sexual mode and may provide a shortcut to your arousal.

A different way of taking responsibility for your desire is to actually start touching yourself sexually, so that you are primed for a sexual encounter with your partner. You could touch your nipples, inner thighs, vulva area in general, clitoris, or the entrance to your vagina. This way you're not putting all the responsibility for your arousal on your partner. Another simple and straightforward way to gear yourself up is to take that erotica you picked up for learning dirty talk and read it out loud to your partner. When you find scenes you both like, try reading those together for ten minutes before a sexual encounter. If any of this section on taking responsibility for your own desire feels uncomfortable to you, remember that this is about giving yourself permission . . . permission to be sexual in new ways, permission to step outside your comfort zone, and permission to enjoy pleasure.

The other side of priming your pump is determining what role your partner has in overcoming your sexual brakes and facilitating sexual desire. What does he or she do (or not do) that helps you get out of your head and into your body? A kiss on the back of your neck when walking by? Whispering how beautiful and sexy you are over dinner? Slowly kissing you like you're eighteen years old again? Gently moving their hands all over your body, instead of immediately touching your breasts or genitals? Or something as basic as taking the time to brush their teeth before they share a personal, close conversation with you? It's advantageous to consider what works and doesn't work and to share this with your partner, so you can be a team in facilitating your shift from your head into your body. Your partner is not inside your head and body, so specific and concrete examples are going to make a big, positive difference in this conversation, even if that feels awkward. Remember to breathe through the awkwardness and know that you are strong enough to handle it.

Who's Your Sexual Archetype?

Do you freely express your sexual personality in the bedroom? Do you have fun and lose yourself in the moment? Are you able to be who you want to be? If your answer to any of these questions is "no," consider who *does* embody the energy of the kind of woman you want to be sexually. A fantastic way to play with your sexual identity is to choose a sexual archetype. An archetype is a type of person who we all recognize and understand, such as the Mother, the Healer, the Teacher, or the Warrior. If you were asked to be "the teacher" in a play, you could do so because you know the set of personality traits commonly associated with that role. I expand on this concept of archetypes to include sexual archetypes that can help you grow in your sexual expression.

Typical archetypes connected to women's sexuality

include the Goddess, the Seductress, the Girl Next Door, or the Whore. But I like to empower clients by extending their choices to cultural icons or personal friends, and to images outside of the limited mainstream sexual depictions. Which woman has a sexual energy that resonates with you in a way that you would like to embody? Perhaps a movie star, a book or television character, or a musician? Or do you have a friend or acquaintance who represents sexual authenticity to you? Who do you think of as living in their body in a way that feels sexually empowering and sensually present to you? I've had clients choose Hollywood stars who you might expect, like Beyoncé, Catherine Zeta-Jones, and Julianna Margulies in *The Good Wife*, but also less traditionally "sexy" depictions, like the character Lily in the show *How I Met Your Mother*.

Now get specific about what qualities that woman possesses that you would like to cultivate, and try to bring those qualities into your sexual encounters. For example, the client who chose Catherine Zeta-Jones channeled this star's smooth, calm presence any time she felt rushed or worried. Whether hurrying to a meeting at work or feeling anxious about how long her body was taking to orgasm, she would ask herself (and answer): *What would Catherine Zeta-Jones do? She would slow down, feel confident in her body, and know that she was fine. And I am fine.* My client knew that she didn't *really* know what Zeta-Jones would do, but she could still embody what she felt when she watched Zeta-Jones.

Although doing this might sound like roleplaying, the energy is different because here you are developing comfort with previously unexpressed parts of yourself, with the intention of integrating them into your sexual personality.

This is not performance, but an experiment to discover new yet authentic sexual expression. I'm suggesting that you tap into a sexual attitude that resonates deeply with you but that may have been blocked or never developed. Give yourself permission to have fun in the exploration and expression of new facets of your sexual being.[97]

Initiating Sex

Who initiates sexual interactions in your relationship? If there is any sexual unhappiness in a relationship, initiation tends to be a touchy topic, fraught with discomfort or feelings of rejection—because initiating a sexual encounter can feel vulnerable, especially if you've felt rejected by your partner in the past or if you're afraid you don't know how to initiate. I've heard women who had lower levels of desire than their partner share this reason for avoiding sexual initiation: "What if my body doesn't turn on all the way and I want to change my mind?" This is an excellent question, and quite a valid concern. They're afraid of feeling like they have once again disappointed their partner. However, there are some clever ways to initiate sexual interactions that give you both some wiggle room.

I worked with a queer couple in their late twenties in which one partner had previously been in therapy because of childhood sexual abuse. Sexual encounters still felt inappropriate and uncomfortable to her at times, let alone the thought of initiating. This meant that her partner was always the initiator, which was also

---

97   This section is adapted from my blog post "Is Wonder Woman Your Sexual Archetype?" posted on July 19, 2013: www.drjennsden .com/blog/2013/7/19/is-wonder-woman-your-sexual-archetype.html

problematic, because it could evoke a sense of obligation that was similar to what she had felt during the abuse. Clearly this was a complicated and sensitive situation. I suggested that instead of verbally requesting sexual intimacy, they try using an object to signify potential interest—for example, taking a particular figurine or knickknack in their home, and moving it to an obvious place for their partner to see. Once the other person saw it, they had thirty minutes to approach and discuss how they were both feeling about intimacy, with no obligations or expectations. The goal was to reduce the pressure on both sides around initiating or feeling rejected. The strategy gave them both time to respond instead of react, and to gauge their sexual interest. It helped reduce sexual anxiety on both sides, as they could have a mindful and compassionate conversation about it.

Other tools to consider for initiating intimacy include a stoplight analogy (red/yellow/green) to indicate interest level, or a scale of one to five to indicate how sexual you each feel. These tools allow you time for a mindfulness check-in with what's going on for you in the moment, whether your body and mind want to feel sexual, and how emotionally close you feel to your partner. The thirty-minute lag time can be helpful with these tools, too. Use that time to pull out the Triangle for a body and mind check in. Observe your thoughts and beliefs about your body and your partner's expectations. Remember that they are your *interpretations* and not necessarily *facts*. Are you feeling excited, scared, tired, disconnected? And where do you feel those sensations in your body?

If your partner has just expressed that they are a "green" for a sexual encounter, using the stoplight analogy might look something like this: If you're a definite "no," then say *red*. If you're definitely a "hell yes," then say *green*. But like I said, don't feel like you have to answer right away. If you think you'd like to be physically close, but you're not sure if you feel up (mentally or physically) to sexual play, say *yellow*, and consider what you and your partner could do to potentially turn it into a green. Such systems require the development of a nuanced understanding of your sexual and emotional energy at any given time, as well as learning how to articulate that awareness to your partner. This may take time to develop. Remember to use all of the activities in this book to help you on this sexual awareness journey.

The one-to-five scale is a more detailed way to delineate how sexual you're feeling. If you're not feeling sexual, but still want some physical closeness, it gives you a way to have your needs met and still say "yes." For example, if you're feeling this way, you can say you're a one, and ask if your partner is game for some cuddling. If you're all in and want a full sexual interaction (whatever that means to each of you), then say you're a five. You can discuss the meaning behind the two, three, and four responses together so that you have a more detailed system that works for you as a couple—this scale is personal and might look very different for every couple. (In the next section, I offer many suggestions for how to get things started in less pressured ways, and you'll find many activities that you could choose to include in your one-to-five scale system.)

I want to give you all permission *to give yourselves permission* to be sexual women on your own terms! This means owning your sexual desires, needs, thoughts, and power without shame. This also means being willing to feel or look silly and put yourself out there in new ways. Give yourself permission to surrender to your sexual and sensual truth.

THINKING OUTSIDE THE SEXUAL BOX

Although options for sexual experiences are incredibly broad, we learn a specific, limited way to "do sex" in our society. Many folks never question the learned idea that there are limited ways of interacting sexually and sensually; but in fact, the ways of interacting erotically are endless. However, in a long-term relationship, the scripted and predictable aspects of sexual interactions can be amplified. Between sexual boredom and our always-aging bodies, it's just smart at any age to start thinking outside the sexual box (yes, I do mean this as a double entendre!). The broader and deeper your sexual repertoire (and your partner's), the more sustainable your sexual fulfillment and satisfaction will be in the long run.

How can mindfulness help with this? As you've read, and hopefully have been practicing already, mindfulness is about being present in the moment and bringing greater awareness to the details of what's going on in any moment. "Doing sex" in a scripted way means that you're on automatic pilot. But making a mental shift from business as usual to exploration, play, and creativity allows you to break out of your habits and do sexual activities differently. Exploring new activities may mean that you don't feel as competent, which can feel scary or intimidating. That's perfect. These are the exact kinds of emotions and thoughts you want to observe with your new mindfulness skills, because they mean you're building the courage to address the fears that are holding you back.

Remember to stay present with your fears, breathe through them if it helps, and choose to move forward in that moment. Remind yourself that the second A of mindfulness, Acceptance, means to not judge yourself. Don't judge yourself when you don't know what you're doing, because *nobody* knows what they're doing when they try new things! And don't judge your partner, either. Just show up and give each other a chance to try something new. I even suggested to one client couple that they celebrate any new sexual activity with a fist bump. It's not easy to try new things and risk feeling ridiculous or incompetent. So just the act of doing something new deserves celebration and appreciation. And after the genuine celebratory fist bump, they could discuss what worked and what didn't . . . and if it sucked, for one of both of them, it was okay to laugh and say, "We will never do *that* again!" You can make a mental shift from heaviness and fear to lightness and play.

Setting the Sexual Mood

You can also make shifts around the conditions under which you approach sexual activity. What time of day are you usually sexually active? Is it before bedtime? This is the standard for many couples, which is unfortunate. Many women feel exhausted at the end of their days; they just want some downtime to be quiet or self-nurturing. They want time with no responsibilities or obligations, and sex can unfortunately feel like another chore. Sleep is important in its own right, as we are a habitually sleep-deprived nation, and lack of sleep leads to all sorts of negative effects, not the least of which are stress and irritation with our partners. Therefore, creativity about when you have sexy time is important to creating sustainable sexual intimacy. Is there any chance of getting up even twenty minutes earlier some mornings? Or scheduling an occasional afternoon delight during lunchtime? Or a leisurely morning or afternoon during the weekend, when the kids are still at a sleepover? If this concern about sexual timing resonates with you, this is a valuable conversation to have proactively with your partner, and it may lead to some creative compromises.

Changing your sexual schedule is one way of thinking outside the box to create conditions that will optimize your desire for sexual activity. Along those same lines, here's another question to consider: What positive smell makes you think of your partner? Perhaps something you used to bake together? The lilacs that were blooming the summer you first fell in love? The smell of the gum they were chewing to freshen their breath for your first kiss? Or the smell of their perfume or cologne? When I began having boyfriends, in late high school and college (as I said, I was a late bloomer), one of the popular colognes of the time was Drakkar Noir. My earliest sexual experiences of desire and arousal with a man were connected to the smell of Drakkar Noir. More than twenty years later, if I pass a man walking down the sidewalk wearing this cologne, I feel nostalgic and a bit turned on. It may not sound sophisticated, but the way our brains hardwire smells to specific emotions is.

So how can you use this to your advantage? Once you identify a scent, ask your partner to bring this scent back into the picture, and see if it starts to naturally stir your desire. You can also create a new scent that you positively attach to desire and your partner. For example, if they have a new cologne, grab that bottle and sniff it while fantasizing about them or masturbating. Or ask your partner to wear it when you're feeling particularly aroused. This is a direct route to wiring your desire and arousal to the smell of your partner. And a perfect example of thinking outside the box.

Reconnecting with Just Physical Touch

If you have not had sexual interactions with your partner in a long time, and one or both of you feels that sex has become strained, it can be helpful to first start with physical closeness that has no sexual expectations. A simple yet powerful way to connect physically is with what I call a Melting Hug. At least once a day, when you're walking past your partner or when you're joining them after being away, share a longer hug with five deep breaths. Synchronize your breaths, so that with each exhale you feel your chests melting into each other. This may feel contrived or stiff at first, but give it a chance. The physical touching and deep breathing as a synchronized activity can serve as a sort of sacred reconnection each day, as you choose to slow down together while in physical contact. I know couples who love this activity and look forward to this daily experience. I know others who are split on their opinions about it, but the dedication to physical connection helped them eventually feel greater intimacy.

One reason you may be struggling with sex in your relationship is that one or both of you carries expectations, which create pressure and a fear of disappointment (as discussed in the section Giving Yourself Permission).

A vital component of regaining sexual ground is creating spaces that are about exploration and fun, with no end goals beyond that. This is the difference between *doing* and *being*. The actual *doing* in these activities doesn't matter as much as the energy that you bring to it—your *being*. Who do you want to be in these interactions? Do you want to be heavy, worried, resentful, or shut down? Or do you want to be playful, creative, silly, sensual, light, and fun? Being mindful of your energy and your intentions will help you remember that you *can* have a choice around this. So for the next two suggested activities, consciously cultivate a lighter mental state of no expectations and no goals.

The first activity is not only fun to do, but fun to say: Happy Naked Fun Time! (Also known as HNFT.) It's easiest to explain this by breaking the activity down to each word within the name. So first: *happy*. When you're going into this activity, recall the daily gratitudes exercise from chapter 3 and mentally focus on what you appreciate about each other. As mentioned earlier, it's easy to carry a negativity bias, so instead, start HNFT with one or two appreciations. Share something that you appreciate about them from that day—how they dressed, their good attitude, household tasks they checked off the list, or something funny they said. This also serves to open your hearts, which is vital to connecting in intimacy.

Naked is next—yeah! Skin-to-skin touching facilitates relaxation and the release of oxytocin, a bonding hormone. Plus, if sex has become a distant memory, sharing naked time without expectation can ease your transition back to physical intimacy. If being naked feels too vulnerable, then stripping down to your underwear is fine, but do try to notice what fears are surfacing and where you feel them in your body. You can use your new friend the Triangle here.

Now that you're naked and appreciative, it's time to have some *fun*. If sex has become the elephant in the room, fun might also be a distant memory. But HNFT has no expectation of performance or goals. I want you to just enjoy being sensual and cultivate a *being* of playfulness. For some couples, this is playing board games naked; for others, it's doing a silly striptease for each other; and for still others, it's rehashing their favorite memories from the early days of their relationship while kissing and caressing. Your intent is to create intimacy— whether or not that explicitly includes sexual intimacy is up to you.

And finally, *time*. Yes, you must make the time for this! If sensual activity is important, then schedule time for it just like any other priority in your life. This one piece of advice receives a lot of pushback from my clients, because they are holding onto the romantic notion that intimacy time can and should happen naturally. But let's put this in a different context. If your doctor told you that you had to exercise and lose weight because you were at high risk for diabetes, you would probably make scheduling exercise a priority. If you knew your child was struggling to learn to read, you would prioritize tutoring time. Why is the well-being of your relationship and intimacy any different? Scheduling time for sexual intimacy does not mean that there is a requirement for *how* that time is spent. It's just creating space for connection to happen. It can be helpful to set a timer, because without a "goal" or an endpoint, you might not know when it's okay to stop.

So set a timer for forty-five minutes, then forget about the clock and start having some happy naked fun time![98]

The second activity involves consciously using your five senses when interacting with your partner. For each of your five senses—sight, sound, smell, taste, and touch—choose something you think your partner would enjoy. When I've had couples do this activity, they've chosen a wide variety of items to please their partner, such as lingerie or beautiful travel photos for sight; a favorite musical artist or a guided relaxation audio file for sound; scented candles or their favorite cologne for smell; wine, dark chocolate, or cheese for taste; and a massage, feather touching, or spooning for touch. Sometimes people just use what they can find around the house, and other times they go shopping. You should give yourself about forty-five minutes for this activity, and I suggest that you schedule it in advance, so that you have time to prepare. There is no right or wrong way, as long as you're actually putting some thought into what your partner likes. At the appointed time, take turns with your presentation of sensual items, or treat your partner to all five sensual experiences in a row. Just the act of giving, and the separate act of receiving, makes for a nice mindfulness activity. What does it feel like when you're just giving, and paying attention to the nuances of your partner's reactions? And what does it feel like to just receive—is it awkward or decadent? Just as with the hand massage workshop exercise I described at the start of chapter 2, we can learn so much by mindfully separating giving and receiving. Relax

---

98   This section is adapted from my blog post on May 30, 2016: https://www.drjennsden.com/blog/happy-naked-fun-time-getting-back-to-being-physical/2016/5/30

into the moment and continually choose to bring your focus back to your five senses. For couples who feel scared of being sexual again, I always start by suggesting this activity. However, this is a lovely activity for any couple who wants to feel sensual, treated, and connected.

Getting More Sexual

Kissing is a great activity to start cultivating sexual connection. Although kissing can be much more sexual than hugging and other sensual activities, it doesn't require a lot from you in terms of being turned on, and it doesn't have to last a long time. My suggestion here is to regard kissing as a sensual experience without any expectation of further sexual activity. Sometimes I suggest setting a timer for one minute, and if you can kiss and get lost in the moment, then go for it. Other times I suggest kissing to a count of ten, although the act of counting can distract from sensual awareness in the moment. So my main suggestion is to make sure you have fresh breath, and then slowly kiss your partner and explore their lips and mouth for a longer amount of time than you normally would. Without any time constraints, you can hopefully give yourselves a chance to relax into this kiss. If it helps, pretend you're back in middle school or high school, or whenever you first started making out, and just enjoy this activity for the fun and connection it provides, without any other goals attached. Pay attention to any nuances of arousal if you start to feel a little more charged up by your partner.

Okay, so this next activity might sound weird. But remember your choice to approach sexuality with lightness, experimentation, and a sense of humor! I call this "befriending your partner's genitals," and if you feel uncomfortable looking at or touching your partner's genitals, this can be a powerful activity. For example, I had a twenty-five-year-old client who wasn't particularly fond of penises. They were somewhat unknown to her, and she viewed them as things that needed to be taken care of. I suggested that she name her boyfriend's penis (and balls, if she wanted) and start a friendship.

For several weeks in a row, every Sunday morning for a few minutes as they lay in bed together, she had a conversation with "Hugo" (the name she chose). She asked him what he did and didn't like (and subsequently answered those questions, too), knowing full well that this activity was meant to be silly and playful. Her boyfriend understandably felt awkward at first. But once he realized that she wasn't making fun of his genitals, but was gaining comfort with them, he was also able to relax and eventually enjoy the attention. By doing this for a few weeks in a row, she learned to stop perceiving his penis as something threatening or uncomfortable. The fear of being vulnerable in a silly way keeps a lot of folks from trying new things, and this often serves as a block to deeper intimacy. So, as I suggest with all things uncomfortable, just notice what comes up for you, thank those feelings and thoughts for trying to protect you, choose to stay aware of the present moment, and be kind to yourself.

Sometimes two barriers to sexual intimacy strike in the same context. As mentioned previously, I often hear couples express that they don't have enough time for sex. I also often hear that they don't have much energy to bring to a sexual encounter (particularly just before bedtime, as I also discussed earlier in this chapter), especially if it's more than a quickie. One way around these barriers is to create index cards for Ten-Minute Intimacy Time. Sit down with your partner and brainstorm what kinds of activities you could do in only ten minutes. These activities should interest both of you and facilitate physical closeness. They could cover a broad range, from sensual activities, such as cuddling, wrestling, or foot massage, to overtly sexual activities, such as sharing sexual fantasies, masturbating in front of each other, oral sex, nipple sucking, spanking, or even a quickie of your usual form of sexual intercourse. Be reasonable about what you each would feel good about enjoying in only ten minutes and then stopping. Neither of you should feel pressured by the other to continue.

The intent of these cards (and I suggest you write at least ten of them) is to think outside the box to make short periods of intimate time easier and more frequent, with less pressure and fewer expectations on both sides. If you pull a card and it feels like too much at that time, choose another one. But do be mindful if there are certain cards that you continually neglect, and eventually make time for those as well.

One of the most scripted aspects of sexual interactions is the order in which we do sexual acts. Most of us grow up learning some version of the "bases." First base is kissing, second base is genital or breast touching, third base is digital penetration or stroking (at least when I was growing up—now it's oral sex), and a home run is sexual intercourse. This is problematic for so many reasons, from the competitive and goal-oriented nature of the metaphor, to the prescriptive order in which we think sex naturally progresses, to its heteronormativity. But thinking outside the sexual box means that the baseball diamond does not get to dictate our sexual expression if we don't want it to. Hell, we can run around in the stands if that feels more authentic to us! One of my favorite client experiences was working with a couple on how their sexual activity progressed. She explained that she had sensitive nipples, so it didn't feel right when her boyfriend started touching her breasts after only kissing. She felt turned on enough to enjoy nipple stimulation only once they were engaged in sexual intercourse. I suggested that they make nipples "fifth base." She looked at me with shock and exclaimed, "You can do that?" My point here is that you can *always* do things differently, based on your tastes, sexual wiring, and mood.

Playing with Power

If you grew up learning that men and women—everyone—should always be equal (and I hope you did!), or that sex should always be gentle lovemaking, then the thought of dominating or being dominated by your partner might seem odd. But I've been surprised by how many women are excited by this idea (although with the popularity of *Fifty Shades of Grey*, I shouldn't be surprised at this point). What is your initial visceral reaction to the thought of dominating, or being dominated? Do you want to be dominant, the master of your partner? Do you want to be submissive and surrender to their control? Or both? I think that equality outside the bedroom is incredibly important, but playing with power dynamics inside the bedroom can be incredibly erotic.

If this piques your interest, here are three different ways to approach power play:

▸ Add sensation to the experience, or take senses away. This is the mildest introduction to sexual power play and doesn't require either person to step that far outside their comfort zone. An example of adding sensation is using an ice cube. An example of taking senses away is blind-folding. Think about your five senses and how you could add or remove them in a sexy way. Although I found the book Fifty Shades of Grey to have some major consent issues, I loved the scene when Christian Grey put iPod earbuds in Ana's ears to remove her sense of hearing while also coordinating the music to his actions. Any form of playing with our senses in this way can add an unpredictable, and therefore exciting, new component. This kind of creativity breaks from a predictable sexual script and focuses more attention on specific sensual details.

▸ Physical domination or submission. I think this is what most people imagine when they think of power play—specifically, being spanked or tied up. Domination can involve pain if that inter-ests both of you, but please communicate clearly about boundaries and safety. For many folks, though, it's the taking of or surrendering to phys-ical control that is most arousing. This can involve tying someone to the bed, maneuvering them how you want—or having these things done to you. Again, such activities are generally unpredictable and new and therefore, hopefully, exciting.

▸ Mental domination or submission. This could involve the other person telling you what to do, talking down to you, calling you a slut, etc., depending on your tastes. I've found with more than a few couples in my private practice that the women very much wanted this from their husbands, but the men were afraid to step into this role. It felt disrespectful and degrading. Out of context, it clearly is, but in the sexual realm, consensual naughtiness and taboo-breaking can be stimulating. I never suggest that someone do something they feel morally opposed to, but I do think it's valuable to mindfully explore one's reactions to taboo topics in order to learn and grow.

If you felt any tingling of excitement reading my brief descriptions, we might be on to something here. It's important to discuss power play ahead of time with your partner to ensure consent; it should never be assumed that a partner is interested in any kind of power play.[99] Talk through any fears, expectations, or hopes you have for the interaction. Come up with a "safe" word in case you just need to halt everything in an instant—a word that wouldn't normally be said in a sexual situation, but that signals your desire to slow down or stop what you're doing. If power play interests you, I urge you to research resources to learn about best practices concerning communication, setting boundaries, safe word systems, consent, negotiation, and safety practices

---

99 I've been hearing more frequent stories from millennial women about sexual encounters with men who just assume they want to be choked. This is not okay!

with bondage. There is a lot involved in doing this safely and happily!

Also, discuss what kind of energy and feeling you're hoping to create. Be compassionate and playful with your partner during this discussion and remember that they might feel their own trepidation, too. It's up to each of you to notice any embarrassment or discomfort and ascertain whether you want to move through that discomfort and step into the role you've chosen. If you want your partner to play the dominant role, be as clear as possible about how you want them to treat you, and give them clear examples of the confident energy you're hoping they evoke.

The intent behind all of these activities is to think outside your usual sexual box. You want to slow down, be present in the moment, embrace and breathe through discomfort, and appreciate your sexual partnership in new ways. Finding and embracing your authentic sexuality, especially in a long-term relationship, takes continuous mindfulness and courage.

REFLECTION & WRITING

When you think about the word sex, what thoughts and emotions come to mind?

....

....

....

....

....

....

....

....

What is your main motivation for being sexual? Has that changed over time?

....

....

....

....

....

....

....

....

Can you define your sexual wants and needs?

....

....

....

....

....

....

....

*Have you ever gone along with a sexual activity you didn't
really want to do? Why?*

....
....
....
....
....
....
....
....

*Has your training in "femininity" had an impact on how you
behave sexually? Has it been positive or negative? What
would you like to change?*

....
....
....
....
....
....
....
....

*What expectations do you think exist about how you should
behave sexually? What do you do with those?*

....
....
....
....
....
....
....

What was your experience reading the Blocks to Desire section? What resonated with you from that section?

....
....
....
....
....

What would you like to give yourself permission to do or say, or to not do or not say? Do you think you're good at self-nurturing?

....
....
....
....
....

Do you like being creative with sexual activity? Why or why not?

....
....
....
....
....

★ **ACTION ITEM** ★

Choose a sexual archetype (see page 189), write down the characteristics you most want to cultivate, and then spend thirty minutes today consciously moving through the world embodying your archetype's sensuality.

CHAPTER 5

BODY IMAGE

walked into the ocean. The greenish water felt warm for
San Diego, without the usual sting of colder water on
my freshly shaved legs. As I waded farther and the sun
warmed my bare back, the waves splashed up against my
genitals. My bare genitals. I didn't know being naked in
the ocean would feel so . . . freeing. It seemed cliché to
be at a nude beach and think, *This feels liberating*, but it
genuinely felt that way.

I turned and looked back at the red cliffs, and I noticed
the various bodies dotting the shore. An elderly man with
a belly almost covering his penis walked along the shore-
line. A middle-aged woman with large, hanging breasts
and generous pubic hair unscrewed her umbrella from the
sand. A buff young military-type guy watched as a yogi
couple performed naked acro-yoga. Everywhere I looked
I saw completely different shapes and sizes of bodies.
I'd been there for an hour, and it actually felt like a new
normal. We all have naked bodies. Who cares?

My mind briefly flashed back to the end of seventh grade. Matthew, a drummer I knew from band who was a year older, had asked me to be his date for the eighth-grade dinner dance. I had enjoyed bantering with him during the school year but didn't know him well. My girl-friends had become "boy-crazy" that year, but I didn't get it. Instead of excitement, I felt butterflies in my stomach and panic in my chest at the thought of being a boy's date. I wondered what would be expected of me on a date.

I knew I wasn't ready. But saying no meant hurting his feelings, and even worse, he might hate me for it. I almost stayed home from school with my churning gut and nauseous belly. The next day, I asked a friend to deliver the message. When she returned, she said he'd called me a bitch.

A month later, I was in our last band class, goofing around with my classmates and trying to play each other's instruments. I held my friend's violin to my chin, but I could only get the instrument to emit agonized cries. My clarinet skills were useless there. I had moved on to the timpani to try thumping some deep resonating beats when one of the drummers, an eighth-grader about to move on to high school, approached me. He had shaggy blonde hair and smelled of cigarette smoke.

"I heard you said no to Matthew," he stated. I stared up at him, wide-eyed and frozen.

"Well, you're just flat-chested anyway," he mocked before walking away. My face grew warm as I folded my arms over my chest. Until that moment, it had never occurred to me to consider the size of my breasts, or that larger breasts were apparently better.

I shook the memory from my head. *None of that*

matters, I thought, standing naked in the ocean at Black's Beach. *My body is fine. My breasts are beautiful. All of me is fine as it is.*

I grinned and waved to my friends back on the beach. I felt a lightness in my chest, an ease in that moment of accepting and appreciating the only body I have. In that moment, all of the other stuff seemed absurd—the body hatred, the fears, the shame. Alas, I knew that the moment wouldn't last.

WHAT YOU LEARNED

So many women dislike their bodies. Where do our preoccupation with and negative feelings about our bodies begin? From birth, many young girls hear how sweet and soft, or cute and pretty, they are, and learn that their value is in their appearance. When I was learning about sociology and gender as an undergraduate and then graduate student, we often referenced the classic research studies about "Baby X." In these studies, a baby was presented to research subjects (both adults and young children) as a boy, a girl, or sometimes without a gender specified, regardless of the baby's sex assigned at birth. The researchers then studied how the subjects interacted with the baby, depending on the sex label that was shared with them. Some studies found that the subjects were more physically interactive with a "boy," commenting on his strength. But with a "girl"? They were more likely to perceive her as softer or more fragile.[100]

---

100 This study provides an overview of much of this research: Marilyn Stern and Katherine Hildebrandt Karraker, "Sex Stereotyping of Infants: A Review of Gender Labeling Studies," *Sex Roles* 20, nos. 9–10 (1989): 501–522.

The only thing that was different was the research subject's belief about the sex of the baby lying in front of them. This influenced how they thought they should "naturally" interact with that child. In another classic study, parents of newborns were more likely to describe their daughters as beautiful or pretty than they were to use aesthetic descriptors for their sons.[101] It's clear that what seems natural is constructed by social expectations, regardless of actual sex or a baby's behavior.

What's the harm in this? Specifically regarding women and body image, the harm is that from birth, females learn to feel worthy when they are getting attention for being attractive. Being perceived as attractive, and later sexy, is a way to get attention and praise, versus other avenues such as achievement, hard work, intelligence, athletic ability, or wisdom. Like the drummer in my middle school band class, all members of society—from strangers to friends to family to lovers—feel like they have a right to comment and pass judgment on women's bodies. So whether a female wants to care about her appearance or not, it is imposed on her. This insightful quote from the classic women's health book *Our Bodies Ourselves* brings home this point: "For women, life can often seem like a beauty pageant. Throughout every phase of our lives, from childhood to maturity, our appearance is judged and critiqued. . . . We're rated pretty, ugly, plain—or just plain average.

---

101 Jeffrey Z. Rubin, Frank J. Provenzano, and Zella Luria, "The Eye of the Beholder: Parents' Views on Sex of Newborns," *American Journal of Orthopsychiatry* 44, no. 4 (1974): 512–519.

No one has ever asked us if we want to compete in this lifelong beauty contest."[102]

This might not be *that* much of a problem if advertising and media images didn't take it all to a ridiculous level, where emphasis on women's appearance is ubiquitous. Consider the vast majority of images that you see in movies, television, billboards, ads, magazines, etc., and their narrow presentation of women's beauty. The images indicate that young, thin, tall, white women with large-enough breasts are attractive. But even *those* women don't really look like their media portrayals, because their photos are highly airbrushed with alterations to their body structures to make them look thinner and their skin look flawless. Hips, belly, thighs, stretch marks, arms, face, hair, skin tone—all are altered through Photoshop or filters to achieve some ideal standard of beauty. Almost any time a woman is considered sexually desirable in the media, she fits this narrow standard of beauty.

This heavy topic can be reduced to a simple equation for girls and women: Attractiveness = Worthiness. The insidious impact on many females is that they are in a constant state of self-assessment, critique, and "fixing" how they think their body parts look to others. Women are taught to objectively and critically assess their bodies, instead of subjectively enjoying the gift of their physical bodies. Becoming beautiful and staying beautiful as defined through mainstream media does not happen naturally. This takes a lot of time, energy, and money,

102 Nancy Etcoff, *Survival of the Prettiest: The Science of Beauty* (New York: Anchor Books, 1999), 68, quoted in Boston Women's Health Book Collective, *Our Bodies, Ourselves: A New Edition for a New Era* (New York: Touchstone, 2005), 3.

and allows the beauty industry to make billions of dollars each year off of women's insecurities. As we inevitably grow older, the aging process becomes intertwined with our sense of value and self-worth. For many women this creates a continuous battle with their bodies. We each have only one body, and it does pretty amazing things for us. But we are taught to focus on its appearance to others, and therefore on how it is constantly failing to match up to some impossible image of perfection. This brings me back again to the word "madness" and how this is a really messed-up lesson to be teaching to half the population.

These messages inhabit each of our brains and hearts in distinct and personal ways. A while back, I interviewed "Jackie," a thirty-year-old woman who was lovely and sweet, with a layered and heavy clothing style. She dressed and carried herself as if to try to hide from the world. Jackie shared with me how much her mother had struggled with her weight, and how she had hated her body because she believed she wasn't thin enough. As a teenager, Jackie learned that body image concerns were a way to emotionally bond with her mother. After her mother passed away, she continued to embody this familial body discomfort and fear. But through the work of personal growth, she recognized this harmful belief: If she embraced and loved her body, it meant she was disloyal to her mother. In her mind, her commitment to her mother's memory meant that she shouldn't be sexy or embrace her beauty. Acknowledging this belief system and sitting with the accompanying emotional discomfort was her first step in realizing she could make a different choice.

I would be remiss if I didn't specifically address the impact of social media on body image, particularly for younger generations. It's now the norm for many teen girls to repeatedly post selfies to Instagram, Facebook, or Snapchat, where they can literally quantify their popularity through attractiveness based on the number of likes and comments. When you add filters and easy photo editing, it takes the quote about the beauty-pageant nature of life for many young girls to a previously unforeseen level. Whether posing with thong underwear, a bikini, midriff shirts, padded bras, or pouty lips in heavy makeup, younger women are increasingly learning how to objectify themselves. This level of self-monitoring and performance based on appearance and sex appeal accentuates the belief that a girl's worthiness is decided by others.

Body image plays a large role in women's sexual enjoyment and expression. Some research studies have found that if a woman has a negative body image, she is less likely to feel satisfied in her sexual interactions, may avoid sex, and may not want to undress in front of a partner.[103] It's hard to be open to true intimacy when you're distracted with thoughts that your belly is too big, your breasts are lopsided, your stretch marks are unattractive, or your thighs are bigger than your partner's. Fearing judgment of your body means you're not mindfully attuning to pleasure and your partner. And frankly, it's just not sexy for anyone involved.

What about the things you did *not* learn or hear? There are so many positive and empowering messages that you

---

103 Christopher Quinn-Nilas et al., "The Relationship between Body Image and Domains of Sexual Functioning among Heterosexual, Emerging Adult Women," *Sexual Medicine* 4, no. 3 (2016): e182–e189.

could have learned about your body, that could have been emphasized by your parents, siblings, friends, teachers, and media . . . and by yourself. Consider how you might feel if you had grown up hearing messages such as these: *Appreciate your body in all its strengths, abilities, and changes. Learn to listen to your body's wants and desires. Know that your worth as a human is not based on your size or appearance, but on who you are in this world. Unconditionally love your body—it's the only one you've got.* These messages give you the space to be imperfect, to grow and change, and to look and move in a way that matches who you *want* to be, instead of a narrow standard of who you're supposed to be.

What's interesting, and most disheartening, about this topic is that even when we know better, it's still hard to avoid falling victim to this way of thinking about ourselves. I first learned about the danger of these views in my women's studies classes in college. I'm now in my forties and I still struggle with this. That is why I use the word *insidious*. Like I said in the story that opens this chapter, those feelings of full body self-acceptance can be fleeting. Once an idea becomes deeply attached to shame and our sense of self-worth, it can be a lifetime battle to overcome. But it's a journey worth taking.

WHY WE'LL NEVER WIN

This battle for the perfect body is one that no woman will ever win. Even women who more easily match this ideal standard of beauty (some say they won the genetic lottery; I say they won the social lottery) still have a lot of body image concerns. So what about the girls and women who are further from these ideal standards? If you're a woman of color, disabled, unable to afford braces, have a skin disorder, are shorter, have a stockier build, have narrower eyes (and the list goes on), you may not even be considered on the mainstream playing field. This is another example of a kind of societal madness. Some girls and women internalize this madness and forever compare themselves to others. Some, however, have the support to believe and trust in alternatives to mainstream versions of beauty, or to believe that external beauty is not related to their worthiness. Thankfully, we are slowly starting to see a broader range of body colors, shapes, and sizes in our media.

The cards are also stacked against all women as we age. We do not have a social narrative for women who become more beautiful with age, or sexier as they gray. This narrative does exist for men, though, as evidenced through *People* magazine's annual "Sexiest Man Alive" winners. We label women as "letting themselves go" if they don't do the work to present themselves as youthfully as possible, and dyeing one's hair seems to be more the norm than allowing hair to naturally gray. The Hollywood version of "aging gracefully" is getting plastic surgery or Botox. However, the choice to get plastic surgery gets criticized in gossip columns. Chalk this up as another great example of madness, in the *damned if you do and damned if you don't* column.

Our bodies are inevitably aging, and although we can make healthier choices to take care of ourselves, we cannot fight aging or win against it. The multi-billion-dollar anti-aging industry would like us to believe otherwise, though. Almost every part of our body can show signs of aging, and we are therefore encouraged to spend time and money on products and procedures in a futile attempt to stymie this never-ending list of changes. This can be a lifelong journey for many women, with each new body change bringing about new despair. That's why, when I have the opportunity to work with a young woman on her negative body image, I offer gentle insights into how the struggle only gets worse with age. And I present her with the empowering perspective that *in this moment* she has the unique opportunity to alter the path of her future body angst. The sooner she befriends her body and creates a new, more loving and accepting relationship, the happier she'll be in the long run.

The only way we win this battle is by not playing the game the way it's presented to us. It is possible to shift to a new paradigm of thinking. Self-criticism does not motivate us to perform self-care in a sustainable and loving way. It reduces creativity, appreciation, self-efficacy, sexual pleasure, and our ability to trust ourselves, listen to our bodies, and be healthy. Instead of hating our bodies, we can learn to love and appreciate them as they are. Instead of fighting every sign of aging, we can mindfully study our reactions to them and learn what they mean to us. Instead of trying to fit in with someone else's standards of beauty, we can acknowledge the visceral discomfort of shame and the mental discomfort of questioning our worth, and then feel kindness toward our reactions to the madness messages. In a nutshell, we can be mindful and compassionate towards our suffering. It might sound dramatic to use the word "suffering," but disliking ourselves and carrying continued fears about body judgment from others *is* emotional and spiritual suffering.

Once you acknowledge this as suffering, you have a

choice about what you can do. You can choose a kinder and gentler path. Imagine that you're watching a movie about a woman's life, from a little girl at age eight to a dying woman at age ninety. All her life, she battles with her body, weight, appearance, and self-worth. Despite achievements in life and hard-earned wisdom, dedication to her work and to helping others, generosity and kindness in her personal relationships, and making a positive difference in so many lives, she could never be happy and accept herself as she was. Wouldn't that be a heart-wrenching movie? Wouldn't you want to yell at the screen: "But you're amazing and so beautiful! Your value is so much more than your appearance! You've been kind to so many people and improved their lives!"? But . . . do you say those same things to yourself when you're berating yourself for your looks? Probably not. This is the true-life movie that you, like so many women, may live in. And this can heavily impact your ability to be openly expressive in your sexuality.

FROM SHAME TO STRENGTH

What much of this comes down to is a deep sense of shame. It can be shame that you've gained weight, or that you can't lose that baby weight. It can also be shame that you're too thin and not "womanly" enough. It can be shame from a comment a sex partner made about your pubic hair when you were nineteen years old. Whatever the aspects of your body you may be displeased with, fundamentally, shame stems from the belief that your body is not worthy enough or lovable enough the way that it is, and that you may be rejected for that. It is achingly sad that so many women bear this weight each day. We rarely like all of the parts of ourselves, emotionally or physically, as I mentioned in the Introduction in my personal story about realizing in a women's workshop that there were parts of me that I didn't love.

You've probably read enough about mindfulness at this point to see that using mindfulness techniques is a powerful way to choose to do something differently. It takes a daily practice to begin the process of retraining your mind to accept your body and view it with appreciation. It took many years for you to build the strong neural pathways that trigger negative body image, and it will take consistent, compassionate effort to create alternative neural paths.

I have a few suggestions for you if this chapter has resonated with you. The first one is to consciously focus on grateful thoughts about your body. Write a list of fifteen things you appreciate about your body, including your strengths, what amazes you, what you're happy about. Don't limit yourself to thinking just in terms of general appearance, but also consider the strength of your body and its capabilities (e.g., something like even getting out of bed this morning). Think about your athleticism, power, how you move or dance, your overall dexterity, sexual abilities and pleasures, as well as details like your hair, eyes, curves, or nipples. Whatever you write down, it's all good.

Notice whether you're thinking "yeah, but . . ." while adding items, and mentally dismissing them because you don't believe they are 100 percent true. For example, perhaps you think of adding "I have beautiful eyes" to your list, but then you don't because you think of all the possible criticisms (you have new wrinkles at the corners of your eyes, darker circles from lack of sleep, etc.). This is a great time to whip out the Triangle and get clearer on why you're afraid to own fifteen positive traits. It might take a little while to compile this list. When I've led this activity in women's workshops, the women quickly realized that it was easier to list their supposed flaws than their admirable strengths. Unfortunately, we've been trained to focus on the negative aspects of our bodies, and without mindfulness and self-compassion, we remain stuck there. Once you've compiled your fifteen items, it is important to post this list in several places in your home or car (and keep adding to it!) so it stays fresh in your mind. Every time you see the list, pause for a few moments and read through a few items to revive these positive self-thoughts.

In the Informal Practices section of chapter 2, I recommended the positive flip switch exercise (page 93). I'm going to apply that exercise here and take it up a notch by suggesting that you take one of those positive fifteen things and turn it into a mantra. As I mentioned previously, a mantra is a phrase that you repeat, and in my simplified teaching of mantra use, it is a personal phrase that feels powerful and grounding. Mantras can give us strength and focus when we're working through tough topics. You can use a mantra when you notice a triggered pattern and want to choose a different path, or as part of a daily positivity routine.

For example, when working with a young woman struggling with body image concerns, I might suggest a mantra of *I appreciate that my body is strong.* She could then use this the next time she thinks her thighs are too fat, her breasts too uneven, her nose too big, etc. Or she could choose a more specific one, like *I appreciate that my thighs are powerful,* or *I appreciate that my body gave birth to a beautiful baby.* This is a mindful shift from objective body evaluation and critique to an internal appreciation focused on strengths.

A general mantra that a friend in her forties adopted, based on my idea of the movie about a successful woman distracted by disliking her body her entire life, is *Do I want to be old and have lived hating my body my whole life?* We discussed how that self-hate is such a waste of energy and misuse of the only precious life we each have. As you'll recall, I don't suggest using absolute statements such as *I love my body just as it is*. I tell folks to find something that feels "true" so they don't have that little inner voice acting out and saying *Bullshit!* Being on the *journey* or *path* to achieving a goal is generally more realistic and palatable.

I also want to specifically address folks who are dealing with disability or chronic illness or pain. You may legitimately feel that your body is *not* strong or believe that your body is betraying you. These are heavy beliefs and emotions to carry on top of the already impossible ideals of physical perfection. While each day might feel like a physical struggle of sorts, there are also always innumerable aspects of your body that are functioning well. I know this, because you're sitting and reading this book right now. These might include that your chronic back pain has lessened, or that you have 20/20 eyesight, or that your body is responding well to new medications. And to live with chronic pain or a disability in our society can require quite a bit of emotional resiliency. You might not think of emotional resiliency as "physical," but it is—your neural pathways support you in being emotionally stable. That is definitely a strength. The most powerful appreciations always reside in the details of our existence.

Let's put this into action. Every time you notice yourself thinking shameful or negative thoughts about your body: 1) Acknowledge the thought, 2) Consciously choose to shift your focus and energy to one of the items on your list or to a general powerful appreciation about yourself, and 3) Turn the item or appreciation into a mantra and write it down. This is a continual mindfulness activity of observing what you're thinking, choosing to shift your focus to something different, and creating a powerful reminder based on that. Keep this list and your mantras in front of you so you can use them as ongoing personal growth and happiness tools.

Since shame is so ingrained and ubiquitous in our society, you may find it difficult even to notice the ways in which you judge your body. And you have to be aware of the negative thoughts before your can mindfully shift your focus! If you're having trouble recognizing the body-shaming messages you're sending yourself, one strategy is to take note of any shaming messages you may send *others*. One of the ways that we unwittingly maintain our judgmental culture is in the negative comments that we make about other women's bodies. This is very common when we're growing up, especially in high school and college. You may have a female friend who is always making negative comments about what other women wear, how they dress, or how someone has gained weight. This is the kind of gossip that tabloid magazines and websites thrive on. But it is indicative of someone who is not happy with themself. If we were truly okay with ourselves, we wouldn't need to judge or be catty about other women to build ourselves up.

This type of behavior can illuminate our judgments of ourselves and our own insecurities. And it brings us all down. I suggest noticing your judgments of other women for their appearance or their sexual expression, and use that as a mirror to ask: *What am I not comfortable with in myself? Why does it make me feel better to judge her?* Sit with the discomfort of whatever comes up, and perhaps do some compassionate journaling on your insights. Then pat yourself on your back for having the courage to reflect in such a way.

The Beauty of Your Genitals

As I discussed in chapter 1, negative body image can also include a woman disliking the appearance of her genitals. If this is something you struggle with, I have two specific suggestions. The first one is to check out the photography book called *Petals*. This is a coffee table book with close-up, sepia-toned photographs of vulvas.[104] It may be shocking at first, since we rarely see vulvas like this. But the most shocking thing—in a positive way—is the incredible variety of the vulvas. As cheesy as it may be to say, they are kind of like snowflakes, with no two that look alike. If you're not sexually involved with other women, you may never get to see vulvas up close, let alone see them presented as beautiful body parts. I once showed some of the *Petals* photos on the projector screen to a college class I was teaching. The students were stunned into silence, and in their writing assignment afterwards, many women shared that it had never occurred to them

---

104 I highly recommend this 2003 book by photographer Nick Karras. I use it often, but I do have an issue with the fact that most of the vulva hair has been shaved or highly trimmed. This was the choice of the women who posed, and it represents this cultural time period when public hair is considered unattractive or unsexy.

that their genitals could be considered attractive. (While I'm telling you about the original *Petals* book here, there is also a follow-up, color version with educational tidbits included.[105])

This next suggestion might sound terrifyingly vulnerable, but give it a chance. Have you ever experienced a vulva massage? It's like a massage to any body area, but in this case, having someone use their lubricated fingers and hands, with light to heavier pressure, to massage your vulva. This could include the inner thighs, outer lips, inner lips, external clitoral region, vaginal opening, and perineum. The basis of this massage is external touching without penetration, so discuss this with your partner ahead of time to ensure agreement. Once you get going, there's nothing for you to do but receive the touch and give kind and relevant feedback about what feels best.

It's okay if you don't feel turned on during this massage. It's also okay if you do. What seems to surface most for women is shame, embarrassment, or a fear of judgment of their genitals. So it can be helpful, too, if your partner is willing to share what they specifically like or appreciate about your vulva, such as the color, shapes, or even a cute mole. This can feel incredibly intimate and vulnerable, and when I give this as a homework assignment to clients, it's common for them to avoid it at first. But this level of vulnerability and presence, and the self-acceptance that it fosters, is foundational to reinventing sex for women.

If you think that this activity would be valuable for you to experience (or even just pleasurable for you!) but

---

105 This one is called *I Love My Petals* by Sayaka Adachi and Nick Karras. And I'll let you in on a little secret—I posed for this book! But I'm not telling you which one I am.

you feel wary about trying it, use the Triangle and spend five minutes delving into your fears and discomfort. Don't forget to accept what you notice and have compassion for your discomfort. Check in and see if you have the courage to move through this discomfort to a place of greater self-acceptance, and then move forward with the exercise.

Healthy and Mindful Eating

One topic that I don't often hear addressed within the feminist body empowerment narrative is that of healthy eating. I believe that mindful living is highly connected to what we choose to put into our bodies. But this can be a sticky area, because often what is prescribed as healthy eating is actually a thinly veiled reproach, urging us to stay thin and conventionally attractive. I think that healthy eating is a balance between three things: eating what is indicated in the latest research as good fuel for your body (e.g., a variety of natural foods in their whole forms), eating what makes your body feel good after consuming it (e.g., food that gives you energy without making you feel bloated or depressed), and eating in a mindful, appreciative, and thoughtful manner (refer back to the section Mindful Eating in chapter 2, page 90).

This isn't to say that we can't enjoy tasty treats—I, for one, have a total sweet tooth. But I think it's valuable to ascertain your motivations for your food choices (e.g., hunger versus emotional fulfillment or boredom), to savor the taste in the moment (instead of feeling guilt or being distracted), and then to pay attention to how your body feels afterwards. Developing mindful awareness overall means that we can study our patterns around mind and body and find out what actually makes us happier and more harmonious in the long run. Post signs around your eating areas as reminders to slow down and appreciate your nourishment.

Move in Your Body

Our bodies can do a lot of amazing things, but as I wrote previously, if we just pay attention to the way they look and our dissatisfaction with that, we get stuck in a downward spiral of shame and negativity. Using your body and moving in your body, in conscious and intentional ways, can be a tool to override negativity. If you don't already do this—through activities like sports, walking, running, weight lifting, martial arts, yoga, or dance—consider what kinds of movements you might enjoy. Whether for exercise purposes or not, freely moving in our bodies helps us get out of our heads and be present in the moment and aware of our bodies.

One of my clients who struggled with body shame and overeating just had to get outside and take a lunchtime walk around her building to remember how good it felt to move. There's a funny thing that seems to kick in to our brains when we take the time to exercise—it creates a sense of agency in our ability to enact positive change in our lives and reinforces the belief that we are important enough to be cared for. Even a simple exercise like stretching our arms for ten seconds while gently shifting to each side is an example of feeling good through movement and attuning to our bodies. The more we feel good through movement, the more we can recognize and appreciate the gift of our bodies.

Monitoring what we eat and how much we exercise can have harmful motivations, though. Several years ago I conducted a women's small-group workshop in a cute outdoor restaurant on the topic of intimacy and self-knowledge. I was discussing the insidious aspect of body image and how we don't realize how often negative thoughts about our bodies, or a fear-based need to control the appearance of our bodies, influences our choices. One of the women proudly shared how she rarely thought about body image and was really good about self-acceptance. I asked about her exercise routine, and without irony she seriously replied, "Oh yes, I exercise at the gym every day. I could never miss it." I gently probed to unearth her motivations, such as athletic enjoyment, stress reduction, or weight management. She shared that she was quite disciplined in her exercise regimen and unhappy with herself if she missed it because she felt "yucky" and heavy. She didn't mention doing so for health reasons. In the end, it became clear that she seemed good at self-acceptance because she mentally and physically kept herself in alignment with societal beauty expectations. Her fears around weight and appearance had become normalized.

Even if you love sports or exercise, this doesn't mean that you can't bring mindful awareness to your motivations for exercise or eating healthier. Do you exercise because you want to be healthy, live longer, reduce stress, feel good about yourself, or have fun? Or because you are disgusted by your body and fear you must constantly monitor it? The latter is motivated by negative belief systems and can lead to unhealthy behaviors.

I hope that it has become clearer how much shame can run the show regarding body image. Shame feels heavy and makes us want to hide from the world, but appreciation and strength feel uplifting and motivating. The more that you are aware of what you've been taught and how you've internalized those messages, and the more you choose to have compassion for your suffering and the suffering of other women, the more we can all create a new version of sexy.

THE NEW SEXY

We all come in different glorious shapes, sizes, colors, and ages. We know this. And there are variations on what is considered sexy, based on upbringing, ethnic background, and the cultural values that we've been exposed to. But we don't necessarily know that it's possible to believe we are enough exactly as we are, or to feel sexy no matter our appearance. We aren't told that we are sexual, and can be sexy, any way that we look. The negative messages to the contrary can have a huge effect on our sexuality and comfort with being naked around another person. All of the suggestions I've already mentioned are helpful ways to start feeling sexy. Below is a suggestion to take it even further.

First, start by writing down your definition of "sexy" and where you learned it. Does your definition feel empowering or disempowering? What does *sexy* look and feel like physically? What does it mean mentally and emotionally? When do you feel sexiest? When do you feel least sexy? Throughout this writing process, be kind and gentle while also giving yourself permission to dig deep. Notice any self-judgments that surface, and the accompanying bodily sensations. Consider whether you feel open and light and appreciative in your heart center, or tight and protective. Use this process to get clearer on what aspects of your definition come from self-love and acceptance (open-heartedness), and which ones come from impossible societal expectations or shame (closed-heartedness).

Now consider what you think would help you feel sexy more often, and what is a healthy path to cultivating that feeling. Can you tweak your version of "sexy" to include an acceptance of you and your body as it is? Does it involve your physical, mental, and emotional strengths? Do you know a woman that you admire who is outside the norm of "standard beauty" yet embodies sexual confidence? Take some time to reflect on all these questions and write about how your version of sexy can feel both authentic and empowering right now.

Next, plan a gathering with your like-minded girlfriends to create a new version of sexy for each of you. Make it a party—and why not? Creating and owning your sexiness is a reason to celebrate. Ask your friends to answer the questions from the previous two paragraphs, and then everyone can share their answers. This is a valuable practice in vulnerability, overcoming shame, and learning from each other. You may be surprised by the variety of nuance in what feels sexiest to your friends. Discuss how your definitions have changed as you've aged, and how factors like pregnancy, long-term relationships, media images, and jobs are relevant to your definition of sexy. As the facilitator of this gathering, make sure you're maintaining a safe, nonjudgmental space so your friends can freely express their beliefs and experiences without shame or repercussions.

Now, go old-school art class, and break out your paper and pens, markers, or crayons so each woman can draw words or images that represent a new version of sexy. This is not about artistic ability, but about organic fun and mindful self-expression. The goal is to explore the many components of sexiness that you've already covered in your journaling, and perhaps some new ones you hadn't considered, such as attitude, confidence, strength, talent, sensuality, eroticism, clothing, creativity, movement, appearance, and of course, mindfulness. If anyone is struggling to let go and be creative, gently guiding them through the Triangle process might be helpful, if they're interested.

Finally, invite each woman to list three things she'd like to actively integrate into her life to create and embrace this new version of sexy. Make this a concrete list, with deadlines, and assign accountability partners in the group to check in with each other on a specified date. This might sound like overkill, but generally the only way we make substantial personal change is to start with baby steps and have accountability (more on this in chapter 7). Go around your group and have each participant share their art piece and at least one of the items on their list. It can be powerful and inspiring to do this as a group, because you get to support each other in your unique standards of sexiness, something we rarely see or do in our society. If the group energy from this discussion feels right, schedule a follow-up party to check in with each other, or even better, a day adventure or night out where you put your new definitions of sexy into action.

I want to make a special note about attitude and confidence regarding sexiness. It may be cliché to say that sexiness is about confidence, but there is a lot of truth to that statement. People respond to us differently when we carry ourselves with confidence. I remember years ago when I somewhat sheepishly tried a confidence exercise that had been suggested to me. I was at a restaurant with a date, and

I excused myself to walk across the restaurant to the rest-room. While in the restroom, I looked in the mirror and told myself how amazing I was. How sexy, strong, and powerful. *You're the woman, Gunsaullus!* I thought with an internal laugh. As I left the restroom, I held myself taller as I strolled across the restaurant with a confident gait and rejoined my date. Several heads turned as I crossed the restaurant, and my date had greater energy and interest in his eyes when I returned. Could I have made this all up in my mind? Sure. But try it for yourself and see what you think!

I also unwittingly did a "research" study in a bar once. I was out with a group of women for drinking and dancing in downtown San Diego. All of the women were dressed in short or tight dresses and high heels. Me? Not so much. I was dressed more casually, and I was nearing the end of a long-term relationship. I was aware that I would soon be back in the dating scene and expected to play this "femininity" game. My eyes were wandering the bar, checking out men. But in that moment, I was unhappy. Despite knowing that my relationship had run its course and its end was a good thing, at forty years old, I didn't want to play the dating game again.

Instead, I found a cushy, stately chair near the entrance of the room and sat down, taking up a lot of space in the chair. I lounged back, arms open to the side on the leather chair, and crossed my legs with my right ankle over my left knee. Unwittingly, I was demonstrating a stereotypically dominant, confident male posture. I think the societal expectation for me to take on the pretty, passive, stereotypically sexy female role felt disempowering. I decided I didn't care to play that game.

I was surprised and amused by what happened next.

A group of twenty-somethings walked into the room and paused near where I was seated. I perceived a distinct difference in how the women and men viewed me: Several of the women seemed disdainful, while several of the men seemed curious. Then a man from a different area of the bar sauntered over, stood in front of my chair, and began pretending to do a striptease for me. I was initially stunned; this had never happened before. His actions got the attention of some of my girlfriends, who came closer to watch. One of my closest girlfriends sat down on one of the arms of the chair as we glanced with bewilderment at each other. And then another man, who I don't think even knew the first man, started mimicking a striptease as well, undoing the top buttons of his Oxford. I started whooping and hollering and calling for them to take their shirts off. "Show me more!" I yelled, to the cheers of the surrounding crowd. When the moment had passed, my friend turned and asked, "What the hell just happened?" I didn't have a clear answer for her, but I was aware how powerful I had felt by taking on a confident, broad posture. It was clear that others responded to my unexpected energy. My point in sharing these stories is that there really is something to the energy of confidence, even if we have to fake it until we make it.

There's one other note I'd like to make to conclude this chapter. I want to be clear that I'm not saying you should stop wearing makeup or shaving your armpits or dyeing your hair or dieting, unless you already know you want to stop engaging in those activities. What I'm suggesting, which isn't a surprise since this is a mindfulness book, is to bring awareness to the angst you carry about your body image, and to the choices you make about how you spend your time, money, and energy. Be conscious of the choices that you're making and why you're making them.

Many years ago, I was speaking with a woman in her mid-twenties who presented workshops to women on how to be sexy. She was sharing how she prepared herself for her husband when he was coming home. She talked about the ritual of shaving her legs, wearing high heels, and putting on her elaborate makeup. She was presenting this as empowerment for women. I asked her *why* those things made her feel sexy and *why* they were empowering for women. She couldn't answer those questions beyond stating that they made her feel like a woman and her husband thought it was sexy.

Maybe this works for you, too, and feels empowering. Maybe you love the sensual pleasure of shaving your legs, the confidence and strength you feel wearing high heels, or the playful adventure of trying new looks and personas through makeup. But I want to challenge you to question *where* and *why* you learned your version of sexy. Use the top of the Triangle to question your thoughts and where you learned this meaning of sexy. Then integrate the emotions part of the Triangle to discover your fears of what would happen if you weren't sexy in this way. I'm not suggesting that you overhaul all of your beauty regimens, just that you be a more conscious consumer of the messages you've been fed. As I've written previously, realizing that we have choices that we didn't know we had is the epitome of empowerment. Remember that self-hatred is not a motivator for positive change, but compassion, appreciation, and acceptance are.

REFLECTION & WRITING

What's your earliest memory of learning what the appearance of your body means to others or to you?

....
....
....
....
....
....
....

Did you ever hear positive messages about your body that didn't have to do with appearance?

....
....
....
....
....
....
....

Do you recall anyone commenting on your weight when you were young? What impact did that have on you?

....
....
....
....
....
....
....
....

At what age did you first diet? Why?

....
....
....
....
....
....
....

Do you post photos on social media or look at a lot of social media feeds? When you do this, do you feel better or worse about yourself? Why?

....
....
....
....
....
....
....

How do you feel about your aging body? What does it mean to you to grow old gracefully? Does that feel empowering or disempowering?

....
....
....
....
....
....
....
....
....

When do you feel sexiest and why?

....

....

....

....

....

....

....

....

How can you make choices that come from a place of strength and self-love, versus criticism and self-disgust?

....

....

....

....

....

....

....

....

★ ACTION ITEM ★

Try the activity where you walk to the restroom and pump yourself up, then walk back to your table with greater confidence and poise. You can also do this when leaving your car and looking in the mirror, or just before walking through a crowded space. There's no right or wrong way to do this, but have fun, be kind to yourself, and see what you notice.

CHAPTER 6

OUR RESPONSIBILITY

"This is how I came to love my vagina. It's embarrassing because it's not politically correct," I began, as 250 enthusiastic audience members peered at me up on stage. "I mean I know it should have happened in a bath with salt grains from the Dead Sea, Enya playing, me loving my woman self. I know the story. Vaginas are beautiful."[106] The audience laughed as I performed my *Vagina Monologues* piece. I couldn't have guessed this would be my first of ten productions at various universities and community groups over the following years.

One year earlier I had sat in the same university theater with rapt attention and awe, flanked by three of my closest female graduate school friends. *Holy shit*, I thought. *They're talking about orgasms. And periods, women's pleasure, pubic hair, rape—all in public. And some of it's*

---

106 Eve Ensler, *The Vagina Monologues* (New York: Dramatists Play Service, Inc., 2000), 18.

really funny. Before the end of the ninety-minute show I had turned to my friends, whispering, "I want to be up there next year."

Now, a year later, I was up on stage talking about vaginas and vulvas. I had stage butterflies in my solar plexus but also felt a full-body giddiness. I hadn't realized how perfect *The Vagina Monologues* was for me. From funny rehearsals, to evenings spent licking our fingers after making chocolate vulva lollipops, to shared excitement when I met other actresses on campus, I had never experienced such a collaborative and supportive environment. And like all productions of the play, it was a fundraiser for a local nonprofit that supported women who were victims of domestic violence or sexual assault.

I felt pride in being a part of a fundraising movement that brings voice to silenced topics that are especially taboo for women. We became activists around female sexuality. The shows brought people together in community to witness personal monologues, and everyone in the audience wanted us to do well.

Before my monologue, I had peeked from backstage and seen an older woman with tears in her eyes, a collegiate woman sitting on the edge of her seat, and a group of fraternity men confused and surprised that it was okay to laugh out loud about menstruation. Where else could you find this kind of normalization of female sexual experiences— from the mundane to the horrible to the humorous—that was also a celebration of female pleasure?

I went on in my monologue to point to the source of women's body hatred—patriarchy. We learn that our bodies—sexual and otherwise—are to be disgusted and hated. But that didn't have to be our truth, because it wasn't real. And one by one we could take a stand against it to change this cultural pain for women.[107]

* * * * *

We all have a role in changing the state of affairs in female sexuality. Imagine if more of the people who raised and socialized you had been able to work on their issues around sex, facing their shame, embarrassment, or discomfort. You would have been raised with a healthier version of female sexuality and a more positive body image. We have a chance to make substantial changes for younger generations—our daughters, sisters, nieces, students, and complete strangers—by doing this work ourselves. We also have a responsibility to all the male-identified individuals in our lives to teach and create a new status quo of respect and kindness towards women and men. This chapter delves into how we can create an alternative path forward.

WHAT FIFTEEN-YEAR-OLD GIRLS NEED TO HEAR

As part of a personal growth class, I interviewed thirty-five women on their views on female sexuality and their personal experiences.[108] I asked physical, mental,

---

107 I highly recommend reading *The Vagina Monologues* and/or seeing a local production of the play, if you haven't already.

108 I conducted these interviews in 2007, and the women ranged in age from twenty-two to seventy. Most identified as heterosexual, although several identified as lesbian and several as bisexual. One quarter identified as African American or black, Native American, Latina/Mexican/Puerto Rican, Italian, or Pacific Islander/Asian American, and the rest as white. Their religious affiliations, both childhood and current, included Jewish, Catholic, Christian, Buddhist, and atheist. However, the majority described their current beliefs as including some version of spirituality.

emotional, social, and spiritual questions. Two of the questions were particularly relevant to this chapter. I started each interview by asking, "If you could share or teach something to a fifteen-year-old girl about her sexuality, what would it be?" The final question was, "What do you wish you had known about your sexuality as a fifteen-year-old?" I chose age fifteen because it's in the early years of high school, on the cusp between childhood and womanhood. Girls this age may be experiencing sexual desire for the first time. Their bodies are changing, and the societal pressures to be pretty and get attention are in full force.

Several themes emerged in response to these two questions. I'm including many direct quotes from interviewees below, with their self-described demographic information. I think it's valuable to hear, directly from the mouths of women from various backgrounds, what they think we need to be doing differently.[109] See if you can feel the vulnerability and power behind the voices of these women.

Theme 1: Love Your Body and Respect Yourself as You Are

> "I wish I could go back and tell that fifteen-year-old that I was phenomenally beautiful and I had a kicking booty, and I shouldn't be so self-conscious about it." (31, dating a man for eight months, heterosexual, white)

---

109   The demographic information after each quotation includes age, relationship status, self-identified sexual orientation, and race/ethnicity. The quotations are slightly edited for clarity.

"Really respect your body . . . and enjoy it and take pride in who you are. . . . You know if you are naked and you scream and you really enjoyed yourself sexually and there are people right in the room next door, just do it. So I guess that would be sexual empowerment, to feel good about what you think. Not give a fuck." (55, married to a man for thirty years, heterosexual, white)

"I'm embarrassed to say I wish I knew how much power I had because of [being sexual]. I don't know why I'm embarrassed to say that. But I wish I knew how powerful my sexuality could be. *So* powerful." (31, married to a man for four years, bisexual, white)

"The first thing that comes to mind would be reframing menstruation and how it's a glorious thing. And not something to be ashamed of or pretend it's invisible or just all the stigma that goes with that." (31, dating a woman for thirteen months, bisexual, white)

"It would be about honoring her body, loving it and getting in touch with who she is regardless of what anybody else speaks or thinks." (70, single, heterosexual, African American and Native American)

"Your body is your temple, *that* you know. You have to love it and respect it and be good to yourself." (55, married to a man for thirty years, heterosexual, white)

Theme 2: You Can Put Up Sexual Boundaries, or Wait, or Say No

"I would teach her that [her sexuality] is not something that she has to give away in order to feel validated. . . . And that what matters most is that she feels ready for that experience and that she feels that she's connected with and trusts the person that she's with." (39, dating a man for three years, heterosexual, white)

"I'm hoping that another fifteen-year-old would avoid . . . my bad decision that came from wanting to fit in. . . . After all, my friends were having sex and doing this. I would say fifteen is too young to have sex, period. So I'd be more respectful about yourself and your own body first before just following the masses on having sex." (31, married to a man for one and a half years, heterosexual, white)

"When I was growing up it was an important point to say yes, because of the good girl [ideology]. Your job is to make other people happy. You're nice and so you say yes, and you help out. . . . I was told pretty early on, in an argument with my mom, that my feelings didn't count. . . . So I had those years where I felt like I wanted to say no, but I had no permission to say no." (35, dating a man for two and a half years, heterosexual, white)

"I would say number one, sex is not a weapon to be used against yourself or others. That really it is a gift that is meant to be enjoyed responsibly. . . . You don't give it away to someone who doesn't deserve it, big time, you know?" (33, dating a man for four years, heterosexual, white)

Theme 3: It Is Normal to Enjoy Sexual Feelings and Explore

"Our bodies go through changes and we feel things that our parents don't talk about, like when someone touches us, with the goosebumps, or our nipples getting hard, or getting wet. Those are natural; it's what you do with it that is significant. . . . My sexuality isn't because of who I'm with, but it's mine. My sexuality isn't determined by the partner that I have, but it's mine by myself." (44, dating a woman for two years, lesbian, Mexican)

"I wish I knew that it was okay to be a sexual creature, it was okay to masturbate, it was okay to want to explore. I wish someone was bold enough to say in what ways exploring sexuality was healthy and what ways were unacceptable, a.k.a. my brother [touching me]. I didn't know anything and it was all such a big taboo secret that I grew up completely detached from myself as a sexual creature. And yet . . . I know I am a sexual creature. It took a long time of going back and forth between being okay with that (even feeling empowered by it!) and being ashamed of it, to get where I am now . . . which is mostly okay with it!" (39, dating a man for three years, heterosexual, white)

"Find what's true for her, without being afraid of what her mother would think, her boyfriend would think, her neighbors would think 'cause it's not about that. . . . I wish I had that knowledge back then, that it's just about what is true to me." (23, married to a man for three years, heterosexual, Italian)

"It's all right to be a lesbian, gay, or whoever you are. And that we're all God's children, and he loves us no matter what." (63, dating a woman for two years, lesbian, African American)

"That [sex] is okay, it's fun . . . it can be actually one of the most beautiful things you can ever do, you know. . . . It's not this nasty little secret, anything bad, but it's actually a gift." (37, single, heterosexual, Latina)

Theme 4: Overall Sexuality Education and Sexual Values

"I wish I had known and talked about sex in a way that's holistic like we are doing now. In a class or in some way . . . I wish I had a mentor at that age . . . like a little mini Dr. Jenn, like a teacher." (22, single, dates 60 percent women and 40 percent men, white)

"I wish I had known about sexual diversity more, you know, and that there is more than an option of heterosexuality." (32, dating a man for two years, bisexual, Puerto Rican)

"That it might take a while for [your sexuality] to emerge . . . that it's not like the movies depict . . . . They're not really getting, I think, real satisfaction now 'cause I don't think they know themselves and their body. And I don't know if it's a physical, physiological . . . if it's cultural or whatever, but I would just tell them that it changes over time." (40, married to a man for twelve years, heterosexual, white)

"Say 'This is what I like, this is what I don't like,' and so you have to really sort of take charge. And then also as far as protection, I would probably talk about that. It's incredibly important. So I think it all comes back to valuing yourself and taking some charge, just the way you take charge of what you're going to do in your career, or who's going to be your friend." (56, married to a man for twenty-nine years, heterosexual, white)

What resonates the most with me in these women's stories is that many girls are taught romanticized notions of sex and love, and are ill-equipped to handle pressures, expectations, or negotiations around sex. There's a lack of sex education for young women to learn about their anatomy (including the clitoris) and sexual functions and how to embrace their own sexual desire. In its absence, their experiences are confused, shameful, or detached from their own sense of pleasure. It's also clear that few young women are told that they can love their bodies as they are. Or that being attracted to boys or being attracted to girls are both perfectly normal feelings to have. These themes ring true for teen girls today, just as they did ten, twenty, and forty years ago. Our lack of adequate comprehensive sex education did not serve these women growing up, and it's not serving our young women today.

A NEW APPROACH TO SEX EDUCATION

One of the most basic yet important ways to improve girls' views of sexuality is to teach sex, body, and consent education from early elementary school onward in age-appropriate ways, both informally at home and in formal educational settings. We need to teach younger children that they have a right to boundaries around their bodies, and it is not appropriate for others to touch them without permission (even a hug!). As children age, it's invaluable to teach about the myriad of changes—physical, mental, emotional, and social—that girls, boys, and gender nonbinary youth go through. All of this would include a full understanding of human sexual anatomy (including the clitoris—yes, I'm saying that again!) and how the parts function together. It would also include teaching all children that menstruation is not embarrassing, but a natural, normal process.

As children become teenagers, it is so valuable to create safe, accurate, and nonjudgmental spaces for them to learn about sexual functioning, desire, pleasure, gender roles, emotions, empathy, responsibilities, repercussions, and what sex means to various people. In this context, teens could explore their values and needs and learn how to negotiate sexual conversations with others when they are ready. At the same time, let's also teach them about compassion in dating and sexual interactions. Finally, consent—how to give it and how to ask for it—needs to be taught in detail, including talking about the fear of rejection and the general fear of hurting other people's feelings. Most schools and most parents are not teaching their children these skills. Since it may be awkward as a parent, applying the Triangle and being vulnerable and authentic with your discomfort around the topic is a powerful starting point.

Now imagine if mindfulness training were included in sex education curriculums. At a young age, as kids are learning about their bodies, gender differences, and body boundaries, they could also be learning what to do when they feel social shame or embarrassment in their chest, or when they've disappointed their parent and they feel a dropping feeling in their stomach. They could learn how to feel empowered, instead of angered or silenced, in difficult social situations. They could learn how to identify their needs and make responsible requests at the same time they are learning how to be mindfully present with others. All of these skills would assist them through puberty, with their changing bodies and changing social roles. Learning skills like this at a young age would set children up to achieve much greater competence in communication and fulfillment in intimate interactions. You can start teaching all of this to the children and teens in your life.

EMPHASIZE COMPASSION

I presented two sexual health workshops at a Catholic university a few years ago—one for women and one for men. The women were shy, embarrassed, self-conscious, and pious about sexual topics. The men were very different. They joked about Saturday night hook-ups and talked dismissively about the young women they had sex with. They focused on getting what they wanted and having their pleasures fulfilled, laughing as they talked about not even knowing their partners' names.

I was shocked by their lack of compassion for their female fellow students, so I shared with them the session I had with a young female client, whom I tasked with writing down her reasons for having sex in the past two years. (This is the story I shared at the start of chapter 1.) I told them how she began to cry as she realized the main reason she had sex was because it was easier to say yes than say no. I told this small audience of college men that she was an attractive, friendly, desirous woman who enjoyed sex. She liked attention from men. She enjoyed drinking with them. She enjoyed sexual play. None of these things meant that she wanted to have sex in any given moment. But since she could tell that the man she was with expected it, she went along with intercourse to avoid the emotional and social discomfort of saying no to him.

When I finished this story, the men in the workshop were silent. It hadn't occurred to them that a sexy woman who was flirting and sexually interested wouldn't want to have intercourse; that she might have her own opinions about the pace and timing of different sexual activities. Possibly some of them had lost sight of the fact that such a woman was a human being deserving of respect.

Study after study shows that compassion—for ourselves and others—measurably improves well-being.[110]

---

110   Stanford Medicine houses The Center for Compassion and Altruism Research and Education, an invaluable resource for research on compassion: ccare.stanford.edu/research/compassion-database

Compassion can be difficult to practice, though, due to our cultural ideals of individuality, competition, and merit. It can hard to *want* to care about others who we might think are undeserving of our empathy. Cultivating compassion can initially also be an unsettling process, because it requires *feeling* the suffering of others. But it actually feels good to experience compassion, as a sea of warmth washing through your heart area.

I like this succinct definition of compassion: "Deep awareness of the suffering of another coupled with the wish to relieve it."[111] Compassion is not wallowing in your sorrows or those of others. Nor is compassion sympathy or pity; it is viewing all humans as equals. Empathy is feeling what another human is feeling, and compassion is choosing to do something about it. I call it "empathy in action."

Self-compassion can be even harder to practice. Consider your inner thoughts and how they sometimes become focused on your perceived failures or flaws. Self-compassion is making a choice to give yourself a break, accept that you're human, and focus on positive, loving feelings towards yourself—or at a minimum, choosing a gentler, neutral attitude toward yourself. Whether toward yourself or others, choosing compassion is a gift to the world because it means a reduction of suffering.

During the tail end of writing the first draft of this book, I participated in an eight-week "Cultivating Compassion" class. It sounded lovely—meeting once a week for eight weeks with like-minded people to discuss loving feelings and helping the world, with daily

111 TheFreeDictionary.com, s.v. "compassion," www.thefreedictionary.com/compassion

twenty-minute meditations. I was so wrong! As I learned in the class, suffering is at the core of compassion. Compassion is a four-step process: 1) recognizing suffering in others or myself, 2) feeling the emotions that surface (just as in the Triangle exercise), 3) believing that I can do something to ease that suffering, and then 4) acting on it in some way. To develop this skill, we were instructed in the initial classes and daily meditations to focus on the suffering of loved ones. Sounds terrible, right? It was. It hurt. But it was also amazing. Empathy is feeling what another human is feeling (which can hurt), and compassion is choosing to do something about it, even if that is just sending loving thoughts (which feels uplifting). So even though I experienced suffering, I didn't get stuck in the pain or in feeling hopeless.

This might not sound like much, but it is a powerful shift in how we individually respond to suffering and in our willingness to interact with others. The more that we practice compassion in our heads and hearts, the more we're moved to perform compassionate acts when we're actually faced with a real-life situation. I gained an increased capacity to stay mindfully present with the suffering of others, as well as my own. This was unexpected empowerment.

If you would like support in increasing your practice of compassion, I have a suggestion for a daily reminder. Compassion It is a nonprofit that sells black-and-white bracelets with the words "compassion it" on the inside and outside. You'll notice that "compassion it" sounds like "compassionate," as the intent is to take the word and turn it into an action. Start your day with your bracelet turned to the dark side. When you perform a compassionate act that day, flip your bracelet to the light side. The bracelet is a daily reminder to look for opportunities to practice compassion. You can flip it once during the day when you consciously choose to be kind to another or ease suffering, or you can continually flip it throughout the day as relevant.

This nonprofit also distributes red-and-white bracelets for self-compassion. With the amount of mental self-berating I see with my clients and friends, a daily reminder to self-nurture is vitally important, too. This is a wonderful practice in mindful awareness of your inner and outer environments that helps you find opportunities to be kinder.

I started wearing my Compassion It bracelet in the fall of 2013. I like to think of myself as a kind, caring person as I move through my day, from clients to loved ones. And I found it harder than expected to find an opportunity to go out of my way or do something I normally wouldn't do. So I dug deeper and found circumstances I hadn't considered—times to be less selfish, more empathetic to a friend, or kinder to an unknown person on the street, even if I was in a rush. Imagine how different our world would be if each of us made a daily commitment to compassion.[112]

This commitment to compassion is what we need to change the sexual landscape for young women from shame and disconnection to self-love and empowerment.

---

112 Learn more about Compassion It here: www.compassionit.com The bracelets are sold in pairs, with the intention that your first act of compassion is already built in when you gift your second bracelet to a friend. I'm lucky that the founder, Sara Schairer, also lives in San Diego and was my teacher for the eight-week Cultivating Compassion class.

We need to remember what it felt like to be a confused teenager. We need to empathize with the heaviness of sexual confusion and the anxiety of wanting to be seen and liked. We need to put ourselves in the shoes of these young women and know that *our* voice can make a difference for them. Because it can. Girls and young women hear what we say about our own bodies. How we speak about sex, masturbation, consent, love, and women's sexual expression (or whether we're silent about these topics) all has an impact on the next generation. The messages we share verbally with our daughters (and sons) and choose to post on social media all play a role in maintaining the status quo . . . *or* in creating a new narrative for female sexual happiness and empowerment.

CULTIVATE MEDIA LITERACY

We like to believe that commercials and ads don't impact us unless we're consciously paying attention to them. We also like to think that, since we know that most television shows and movies are fictional, they don't shape our values or beliefs about the world and ourselves. But the soup of images and storylines that surrounds us deeply affects our views of the world.

Becoming media literate gives us back some control. Media literacy is the ability to consciously notice and evaluate media messages, including the "hidden messages" advertisers use to persuade consumers. Gaining media literacy skills involves mindfully studying the messages around us, uncovering the belief systems they maintain or create, and assessing how they make us feel about ourselves and others.

To improve your media literacy specifically with

regards to how women are portrayed, run through this list of questions. When you're watching a television show or commercial, playing a video game, scanning an Instagram feed, or flipping through a magazine, consider the following eight questions:

1. Who has presented this image or message?
2. What is the purpose of the content? What are they trying to sell and to whom?
3. What does the content imply about what it means to be a woman?
4. Does the content portray females in a healthy or strong way?
5. Is a female body being used to sell products (e.g., a half-naked woman draped over a sofa to sell jeans)?
6. What deep human want or need does the content appeal to?
7. How does the content make me think and feel about myself? (Use the Triangle to check in thoroughly.)
8. If I feel bad about myself, or less worthy, who benefits and how?

I'm going to walk you through an example, pulling from my early memories. In the 1980s, there was a douche commercial on TV. The douche company presumably made this commercial to let women know about their product and make more sales (questions 1 and 2). In the commercial, a mother and daughter are sitting by a window, discussing how the daughter sometimes doesn't feel so "fresh" down there. It seems that this was intended to look like a real-life discussion about women's discomfort with their vaginal odors (question 3). I'm unsure whether the mother and daughter were presented in a healthy or strong way, although it was a positive depiction of a mother as a safe person for her daughter to talk to about a personal topic. However, their conversation legitimizes the cultural belief that women should be embarrassed about their periods and the smell of their vaginas (question 4). A female body wasn't really being used to sell the product, but they *were* using embarrassment about women's bodily secretions and functions (question 5). If I hadn't already known that douches were unhealthy and unnecessary for women, I would probably have wondered about my own vaginal smell and whether it was offensive to others. I would have worried that any smell or discharge was abnormal. These messages could have appealed to a deep need to belong, triggering a fear of not being attractive to a potential partner (question 6). I definitely would have believed this was a new personal concern, which could have made me want to purchase that product (questions 7 and 8).

It is eye-opening to start asking questions related to media literacy, and alarming to consider the media's impact. It can also be incredibly beneficial to instill these skills in girls and younger women. Every time I've taught media literacy to teen girls, or instructed parents how to teach this to their daughters, it has had a meaningful impact. The young women feel indignant that the media companies are manipulating their emotions, and they feel empowered by their new insights. Learning these critical thinking skills helps cultivate resilience to media images and messages. Because there are so many negative or inaccurate media images and messages about female sexuality, this is an important tool for all of us.

SUPPORT A NEW SISTERHOOD

If we are going to be role models for a more positive view of sexuality, two components are most needed: 1) compassion, and 2) embracing collaboration instead of competition. I've discussed the value of self-compassion for your struggles with sexual expression and body image, as well as compassion for younger generations so they may learn healthy sex and body messages. I want to add to this the possibility of perceiving other women as collaborators, instead of competitors.

In the Cultivating Compassion class, I learned the phrase, "Just like me, this person wants to be happy and free from suffering." You can look at each and every person around you—from your family to strangers—and know this is their truth, just as it is your truth. This is the truth of humanity; we all suffer and struggle with happiness. This phrase is a lovely way to shift into a different mental state and consider the common foundation of humanity. Imagine how differently the college men at the Catholic university would have treated their Saturday night hookups if they had interacted with those young women from the perspective of thinking, "Just like me, she wants to be happy and free from suffering." It likely would have made them wonder what made that particular young woman happy, and what made her suffer. They might have been surprised to learn that their actions could have been part of her suffering that night or the next day.

Recall times when you felt envious or jealous of another woman. Have you ever felt insecure about someone your partner dated before you, or found yourself endlessly making comparisons to other women? We have phrases like "skinny bitch" to refer to a woman who is thin or "resting bitch face" for a woman who isn't smiling and looks angry. Judgment and competition between girls and women is normalized in American society, and can revolve around attractiveness, sexiness, getting attention, worthiness, or having a desirable partner. Indeed, a lot of reality television is based on women in competition being downright nasty to each other. Apparently, cattiness has entertainment value.

In chapter 5, I wrote about noticing when we're negatively judging other women. This is an important place to take a stand with our friends and loved ones. If you overhear someone saying something competitive or shaming about another woman, consider gently pointing out (without shaming *them* in the process) that those kinds of comments bring all women down. It might help to ask them to consider that the woman is just like everyone else, doing her best in life to be happy and free from suffering. Maybe you commonly speak up about racist comments or sexist jokes, or mockery of disabled people. Body-shaming and sex-shaming other women can be addressed with this same kind of voice.

This also pertains to the "my body is worse than yours" game so many of us play. It goes like this: You're with a female friend, and she starts pointing out the parts of her body she doesn't like, and how bad they look. You jump in and say, "You think that's bad? What about *this* part of *my* body?!" With mindful reflection, you can consider an alternative response, such as: "I struggle with liking my body sometimes too. But I know we're both strong, beautiful, and worthy women, and I'd love to focus on that." That might sound cheesy, but that's because it's so different from how we usually respond in such situations. It is a vulnerable, compassionate, and empowering statement; feel free to craft a version of it that feels right to you.

When you're interacting with a girl or younger woman, bring this same mindful reflection to how much you praise her for her appearance or weight. Focus on her strengths as a young woman and the whole picture of what it means to be a beautiful person. Here are some topic areas and examples to consider when giving praise:

- academic achievement
- athletic endeavors or movement
- music and artistic interests
- service activities
- household chores
- a part-time job
- helpful or compassionate approaches to siblings or older relatives
- commitment to close friendships
- passion and inspiration
- unique perspectives
- strong stands on social or environmental issues

There is nothing wrong with complimenting a girl or young woman on her appearance, but be mindful that you're not giving her the message that it's her *only* source of worth and meaning. Wouldn't it be amazing for future generations of girls to be raised to accept and love *all* parts of themselves—body, mind, and heart?

• • • • •

I want to provide a quick review of what I've discussed about the state of female sexuality in our country. Sex education is woefully inadequate. In the cases where it *is* taught in schools and churches, the focus is generally on the mechanics of reproduction and anatomy, fear of STDs/STIs and pregnancy, and "shameful" sexual activities, but rarely on the messy and beautiful emotional realities, or on pleasure. Media and advertising are replete with images of "perfect" women's bodies that are rarely representative of real women. The media also focuses on superficial examples of female sexual empowerment and rarely portrays the beautiful complexity of female sexual experiences. Women dislike their bodies, often spending time, money, and energy on "fixing" their flaws. There is much shame, guilt, and silence around sexual topics, leading many women to think they are sexually "broken." Because there are so few open and honest discussions around sexual health and sexuality, many women end up disconnected from their sexual power. It is still considered taboo for women to take charge and freely explore their sexual pleasure.

If nothing substantially changes, younger generations of women will grow up believing they are abnormal, dysfunctional, or broken. We each have the power to start creating new sexual social norms of acceptance and empowerment. It is possible to have open communication around sex and sexual health. It is possible for women to be authentic as sexual beings, alone and in relationships, through self-love and exploration. We can all have deeper connections and more fulfilling relationships. And it is possible for men and society overall to learn to understand, feel compassion for, and encourage women, instead of pitting them against each other and themselves.

It is possible to bring this new future to fruition by starting with your own sexual journey of mindful reflection, learning, self-compassion, and expression. I recently encountered a meme on social media with the sentence: "In a society that profits from your self-doubt, liking yourself is a rebellious act."[113] You can expand this new acceptance to your conversations with other women and create safe spaces for women to be kind and real. Then you can look for opportunities to spread these messages to younger generations and create a new path forward.

---

113 This quote was originally from a Twitter post by artist and writer Caroline Caldwell.

REFLECTION & WRITING

What do you wish you had known about sex, consent, sexual health, and self-esteem as a fifteen-year-old girl?

....
....
....
....
....
....
....

How often do you show compassion to others? How about compassion towards yourself?

....
....
....
....
....
....
....

Were you ever taught to question the emotional messages in media? What does it feel like to start doing that in new ways?

....
....
....
....
....
....
....

When did you feel in competition with other girls growing up? When do you feel that as an adult?

....

....

....

....

....

....

....

....

....

What would you like the future of sexual expression to be like for younger generations of women?

....

....

....

....

....

....

....

....

....

★ ACTION ITEM ★

Have an open and frank conversation with a younger woman where you both share some struggles you've faced in the past around your sexual beliefs or experiences.

CHAPTER 7

CREATING YOUR
REINVENTING SEX PLAN

Now we're going to really put this book into action. But before we dive into creating an action plan, I want you to reflect on these questions right now.

- ▸ What do I want in my sexual life?
- ▸ How do I want to be as a sexual woman—and why?
- ▸ What in this book most resonated for me and would enhance my intimate life?

Let your answers to these questions guide you as you begin to create a plan. Spend a few minutes right now jotting down this vision of what you'd like your sex life to look and feel like. Consider the energy you want to carry into your sex life moving forward—playful, attentive, appreciative, honoring, open, creative, honest, etc. These three questions tap into what I've mentioned before, which is paying attention to both the *doing* and *being* of how you are reinventing yourself as a sexual woman. The clearer you are about what energy you want to bring into sexual encounters, and the more you practice shifting to that mental and emotional state, the easier it will be to stay committed to your new actions or activities. (To help you find the activities in the book that may have resonated with you, I've included a List of Activities on page 272.)

CONSISTENCY AND ACCOUNTABILITY

Do you know how long most New Year's resolutions last? Not long. Only 64 percent of folks make it to January 31 (and that's of those who even took the time to make resolutions). Forty-six percent make it to six months, and then only 8 percent claim they are successful in achieving their goals.[114] So you are not alone if you've been serious and committed to making a healthy change in your life at some point, but find that goal a distant memory within a couple months. Instead of beating yourself up, though, know that you're in good company with most other people. This means that there is something fundamentally *human* about sincerely wanting change but being unable to stick with it. Creating new habits is very hard, just like practicing mindfulness; the old ways of doing things are already way more efficient in your brain.

I've suggested numerous activities in this book, and I hope many of them have resonated with you. It's up to you now to make a sustainable positive difference in your sex life and relationship. The most important factor in personal growth is consistency. Consistency is created through baby

---

114   This data was compiled by Statistic Brain, last modified December 7, 2018: www.statisticbrain.com/new-years-resolution-statistics/

steps and accountability. Starting small is more sustainable than trying to make a huge change right away. Also, it's important to create a structure around these small changes that lets you practice them every day, or at least almost every day, of the week. This is how you can retrain your brain. Small, consistent changes are how you slowly build comfort around otherwise awkward or embarrassing topics. And this is how you can slowly build a new version of sexuality for yourself and your relationship.

I have designed this chapter to help you create your own daily accountability structure. That being said, it is much easier to commit to something when you've also given your word to someone else. If you've ever had an exercise partner, then you know how much of a boost it provides to your commitment. It's often harder to feel like you're letting someone else down than it is to just let yourself down. As you work on creating a new daily approach to sexuality, it would be amazing if you could give status updates to your romantic partner about your activities, insights, and progress. You could tell them how you'd like to be checked in on and what kind of words of support you'd like from them.

However, depending on the dynamics in your relationship, this could blow up and create problems, or it could end up feeling like a parent/child interaction. If you have a friend or group of women who are also reading this book, that would be ideal. You could set up a schedule for when to check in with each other, setting goals along the way, negotiating through roadblocks, and keeping each other on task.

If neither of these are options, the structure provided here still works well to keep you accountable to yourself.

Something as silly as adding a smiley-face sticker to your calendar each day that you accomplish your intention can serve as a small motivation reward system.

PREPARING FOR ROADBLOCKS

Acknowledging that it is difficult to create new habits, and then being proactive with this knowledge, is what I call "preparing for roadblocks." While we each have our own unique obstacles that get in the way of change, a number of common roadblocks have emerged in my private practice. There are two main themes: lack of consistency and lack of willingness to keep committing. Lack of consistency is more straightforward. A problem that I hear often from clients is that even when they have the best of intentions, they forget. They also struggle with consistency due to scheduling changes (whether their own or family members'), such as vacations, holidays, travel, or sickness.

Overcoming this roadblock comes down to remembering to be mindful of your commitment to being mindful! I suggest that you post notes around your home, workplace, and car. The more you see them, the more your goals will be on your mind. It's also helpful to frequently move your notes around when they start to blend into the background. The other most powerful way to remember to practice mindfulness is to use current technology to your advantage. Set a phone reminder to go off each day at a time when you will likely have some free time, to remind you to check your homework. If you can't do it in that moment, snooze the alarm so that it continues to go off until you've checked your list of activities and have completed your goals.

A lack of willingness to keep committing is a bit trickier to resolve. This block can have many foundations, such as excitement wearing off after a few weeks, the work not really being a top priority, a lack of belief that you or the circumstances can change, or a fear of failing. I think beneath all of these foundations is a desire to get the payoff of personal growth without the hard work. Many people dream about how they would like their lives to be different, but they aren't willing to dig deep and access their grit when it feels hard or uncomfortable.

If this sounds like one of your patterns, I recommend that you do some journaling about what has gotten in the way of personal growth or goals in the past, and use the Triangle of Awareness to access the truth beneath that pattern. Sit with that discomfort and think about what you can do differently when the pattern surfaces again (e.g., do a weekly check-in to assess motivation and remind yourself why you're committed to working on this, or give yourself a reward that is exciting to work toward, or write about your fear of failure each time it appears). We all struggle with change and commitment at times, but this doesn't mean that we can't continually learn new ways to stay on track.

LIST OF ACTIVITIES

Now you're ready to choose what you want to focus on and how often you want to do so. Here is a list of all the personalized activities in this book so you can revisit them if necessary. (Don't forget the Reflection & Writing sections at the end of each chapter, too.) As you review this list, think about which ones would be ideal for you in a daily, weekly, or monthly practice. And remember, there's a reason I'm using the word "practice." It's okay if you don't feel competent or good at these. That's the point of trying new things and giving yourself the compassionate space to practice—and asking your partner for this understanding, as well.

DAILY ACTIVITIES AND REWARDS

Now it's time to create a daily and weekly schedule to keep yourself accountable for all these baby steps you're going to take. Take your list of all the activities you think would help, or that you're at least curious about, and decide whether you want to do each of those daily, a few times a week (e.g., Monday, Wednesday, and Friday), once a week, every other week, once a month, or one time only. I think the most helpful way to keep track of all of this is to create a special *Reinventing Sex* calendar.

Consider adding some kind of reward system to your calendar. Rewards can be mentally helpful for staying motivated. I mentioned already that putting a smiley-face sticker on your calendar every day that you complete your tasks can actually make you feel proud of your accomplishments. When you feel proud of yourself, you are more motivated to stay the course. Building in weekly and monthly rewards can give you a boost, so it would help to make up a list ahead of time of small, medium, and large rewards. For example, say you'd like to do a Melting Hug every day with your partner. At the end of each week, if you've done it five out of seven days, give yourself a small reward. Or if you add a weekly Happy Naked Fun Time to your calendar, when you hit the end of the month and you've done it four weeks in a row, you can enjoy a medium or large reward. You can create any kind of structure that you want around this. Aim for a mix of being realistic about expectations—remember that this reinvention is best accomplished when done in baby steps—but also being willing to push yourself.

When I was first introduced to the idea of rewards, I balked at the notion. Why should I reward myself for something that I should be doing anyway? This attitude, though, isn't helpful, because there are no "shoulds"— there's only what we are or are not doing. I've since learned that I love adding rewards to a project, because it means that a celebration of sorts is built in. I think that celebrating successes, small and large, is a lovely way to move through life. Rewards in this situation aren't meant to be about spending a lot of money or doing unhealthy things (e.g., rewarding yourself with a bottle of wine . . . daily), but about intentionally doing something as a way of patting yourself on the back for creating new habits.

It's nice to appreciate yourself for making and sticking to this commitment to working on your sex life, which we know isn't an easy topic. A small reward could be a vanilla latte the next morning or taking the time for a walk in a beautiful setting. A medium reward could be a massage or a new book you've been wanting to read. A large reward could be dinner at a new restaurant or a day off to read and drink tea all by yourself. What's most important is knowing that your consistency is some-thing to be celebrated, and, when you're in the midst of enjoying your reward, taking the time to be mindful that you earned it and deserve it.

Now, put your activities into a calendar. I'm old-school and like to have printed or handwritten copies of things to carry with me, but creating a calendar on your phone or computer, as long as you check it daily, would be effective. I suggest committing to this kind of structure for three months, because it generally takes about that amount of time to break old patterns and create new ones. Change it up for the second and third months, based on what worked or didn't, and introduce new activities.

I have two additional activities to consider, in addition to the items from the List of Activities that you may have already added to your *Reinventing Sex* calendar. The first is to remind yourself every day that you are a sexual woman. If you're the kind of woman this book was written for, you probably don't feel like a sexual woman every day. That concept probably feels pretty foreign to you. Which is why this is an important part of retraining yourself to be more sexual. I don't mean that you have to *act* sexual every day, but every day I want you to plant the seed in your mind that you *are* a sexual woman, so that you start believing it.

It's hard to behave in a sexual way if you don't believe you are or can be sexual. So this exercise is as simple as setting your phone alarm to go off once a day, and when it rings, spending three minutes either writing about or closing your eyes and visualizing what it means and feels like to be sexual, for you, personally. Does it mean you feel a tingle in your crotch or a heart flutter? Does it mean you feel desired by another? Does it mean you imagine explicit sexual activities? Does it mean that you feel confident and walk taller? Whatever it is for you, jot it down or think about it, and try to *feel* it. Then write or say ten times, "I am a sexual woman." Or, if that phrase feels like too much (as I discussed with mantras), try "I'm on the path to feeling like a sexual woman." This might make you feel silly, and that's fine, because this is all about having the courage to feel awkward and keep moving forward.

The second new suggestion (which is a mix of previous suggestions) is an actual check-in each day with your partner. The intent of these daily check-in is to give you space to be heard and feel valued. For five minutes each day, share your highs and lows from that day. These can be minor or major successes, emotional struggles, mental difficulties, humorous interactions, etc. After you have both shared about your day, share an appreciation for your partner. This could be based on something specific from their day, or overall. This small time commitment ensures you are not ships passing in the night, but are prioritizing deeper connection and understanding. Concluding with gratitude serves as a reminder of the strengths you appreciate. This kind of daily interaction is an incredibly helpful foundation of relationship connection to support you through at least three months of work on your *Reinventing Sex* calendar.

Perhaps the little voice in your head is claiming that you don't have time for these kinds of daily activities. If so, pause to reflect on that thought. Why are all of your other daily responsibilities more important than prioritizing your relationship connection? As you're choosing your commitments for your *Reinventing Sex* calendar, keep your big-picture goals in mind.

WEEKLY CHECK-IN

The *Reinventing Sex* calendar is for you to explore and design your sexuality based on your big-picture commitments; the following weekly and monthly check-ins are a way to explore and design your *relationship* based on your big-picture commitments. You can add this weekly check-in to your calendar if you think it's valuable to have a regular check-in. If you continually create safe spaces to share how strong your relationship is, or discuss where you need to put some extra energy, you don't end up ten years down the road in an unhappy relationship, asking,

"How the hell did we get here?" I see that all the time in my coaching practice, so consider this check-in an insurance policy against splitting up. I recommend check-ins similar to this for all couples, throughout their relationship.

These weekly check-ins are like taking the temperature of your relationship each week. How do you both feel about your communication? Your teamwork? Your sexual interactions? Because these abstract concepts can be difficult to measure, I suggest using a scale of one to ten to quantify them. I offer suggestions for ten potential topics in the list that follows, although you can create an individualized list based on relevant areas in your relationship. Write down these relationship statistics each week for an ongoing record of positive shifts and also areas of concern.

I worked with a couple in their late twenties who both wanted more physical and sexual interactions during the week. He wanted more hugging, random groping, and flirting (in person and through texts), and she wanted more kissing and playfulness at the start of sexual interactions. They started checking in each week on how fulfilled each felt, with a one representing empty, and a ten indicating total satisfaction. Taking their relationship temperature helped set the intention week after week to pay attention to each other's needs and the nuances of how to fulfill them. Quantifying relationship satisfaction might feel nerdy, but this structure is a powerful tool for relationship evaluation and responsibility.

Here are ten factors that might be relevant for your weekly check-in. While many of these factors are inter-related, they each help pinpoint common areas that could lead to your relationship either thriving or deteriorating.

▸ Connection (Did you feel on the same page with your partner this week?)

▸ Communication (How clear was your communication as a couple, and did you feel heard and understood?)

▸ Respect (Did you feel respected by your partner?)

▸ Teamwork (How much did you interact as a team?)

▸ Nurturing (Did you feel taken care of?)

▸ Love (How full was your love bucket?)

▸ Emotional Intimacy (How frequent was your emotional intimacy?)

▸ Sexual Interaction (Did you experience sexual connection?)

▸ Happiness (Did you share joy and happiness?)

▸ Finances (Did you work together around financial decisions?)

It's valuable to set ground rules for the weekly check-in. Ideally you both bring a positive attitude and are kind, gentle, and mindful. Also, get on the same page about what a two out of ten means, compared to a six or an eight. I suggest that a five indicates you felt average and just okay about that factor in the past week—it doesn't indicate a 50 percent failing grade. Write down your numbers separately and then go through each concept one by one. Be kind and truthful and vulnerable. You will learn details about yourself that you didn't know, such as what helps you move from a four to a six on the emotional intimacy scale. Just like all aspects of mindfulness, this exercise is designed for you to take responsibility for voicing your needs and your perceptions, and to show you that your partner has different but equally valid experiences. This is not about directing blame but about approaching your concerns as a team.[115]

To increase your chances of a *meaningful* check-in, don't do this weekly review when either of you is particularly hungry or tired. Also, be careful to not let heated conversations go on for too long. You don't want this weekly check-in, with its potential to make you stronger, to instead create a wedge in your relationship. Agreeing to a time limit for the check-in each week can help ensure it doesn't feel overwhelming or too negative.

MONTHLY CHECK-IN

Similar to the Small Hurts versus Big Hurts discussion in chapter 3, doing weekly check-ins is a way to make sure that nothing small is getting brushed under the rug and ignored until it becomes something big. But I suggest using monthly check-ins as a way to monitor whether any bigger problems and patterns have surfaced, issues that could derail your relationship. I once read that people who checked the stock market every day made worse decisions in their trading compared to folks who stepped back and took a less frequent, more macro view. This is what the monthly check-in is about. What trends are showing up, and are you headed in the right direction? If the weekly check-in is your relationship report card for the week, the monthly check-in is like seeing the guidance counselor for career conversations.

---

115 This section on Weekly Check-Ins was adapted from my article "How Strong Is Your Marriage? A Checklist," first published on The Good Men Project on December 5, 2013: goodmenproject.com/featured-content/j1b-how-strong-is-your-marriage/

If you've ever thought, *Oh my god, my relationship is becoming exactly like my parents' marriage*—and you don't mean that in a good way—then you know how valuable it could be to have a consistent macro look at things. Or, if you're like so many of my clients in long-term relationships who could have benefited from coaching or counseling years earlier, you know how easy it is to keep living life on automatic pilot without pausing to contemplate where you're going. *This* is the place to check in with long-term goals, personal and relationship fulfillment, parenting styles, and whether you're unwittingly reverting back to old patterns.

For example, I was seeing a couple who had been married for more than twenty-five years, and after a year of working together, they were consistently solid and doing well when I saw them. It was a surprise, then, during one session when they came in and shared that in the past month their marriage had gone downhill. They weren't doing their homework and weren't communicating openly like they had learned to do. It turned out that a conversation in our last session had triggered an old sexual fear in him. He started behaving in a rebellious way when they were at parties and events together, and sometimes blew her off. She was understandably hurt and confused. With the use of the Triangle and past knowledge of his patterns, we realized that his fear of failure had surfaced, and specifically his fear of letting his wife down and disappointing her. Because he didn't realize that this was going on, but was instead scared and reactive, he started acting out in immature ways. When we got to the heart of this, and she genuinely shared that she wasn't feeling disappointed or worried about him failing her, he was able to once again bring mindfulness and compassion to his marriage.

These are the kinds of big-picture patterns, reactions from childhood, and sabotaging behaviors that can be addressed during these monthly meetings. I gave this couple an ongoing monthly assignment to check in with whether he was feeling a fear of failure in their marriage and whether she was feeling rejected or ignored by him. I wanted them to learn to nip this in the bud so they could do it on their own after they were done working with me. This is a concrete way to bring mindful awareness—with its vulnerability, authenticity, and compassion—into your long-term relationship.

I recommend scheduling this meeting in your calendars, with phone reminder alarms. It's also helpful to schedule at a consistent time, such as the last Sunday of the month, so that you always know when it is. Because the *Reinventing Sex* calendar is designed to be a month-by-month commitment to new aspects of intimate and sexual development, the monthly check-in also offers a great opportunity for you to reflect on and share your experiences with your chosen activities that month, and for your partner to reflect back on how they have been impacted by your personal growth work.

● ● ● ● ●

You have all the tools you need now to start doing things differently. Your path to reinventing sex won't always be smooth and certainly won't be easy, but I hope you'll give yourself permission to mess up, fall down, get dirty, and keep moving forward. Any small ways that you can find to consistently start integrating mindfulness into your communication, emotional expression, and sexual inter-actions will bring you a greater sense of self-empower-ment and the intimacy you desire in your relationship. I'm proud of you for starting this journey.

CHAPTER 8

FINAL THOUGHTS

PATIENCE & SELF-COMPASSION

I want to remind you to be gentle to yourself in this process. The concepts in this book are hard and require you to unleash your brave energy. They are all about facing your fears and sitting with your deep discomforts around sex. The reactive patterns that you have in place—to run, numb, or distract from uncomfortable aspects of your sexuality—have probably been there for a long time. They've protected you well. This book is asking you to dismantle your alarm systems, yet also stay open-hearted. This all takes time, so please be patient with yourself, and ask the same from your partner. Some changes will happen quickly, because the timing is right and you are ready for them. Other changes will take longer, some even the rest of your life. This isn't a bad thing. This is just the beautiful reality of your life journey.

Some topics will continue to surface as you patiently

pull back layer after layer of that frustrating onion. I hear it from clients all the time and have experienced it myself—that moment when you realize you're facing the same issue you thought you'd dealt with ten years earlier. You *did* deal with it ten years earlier. And now it's here again, with new depths to it. You're ready for it in a new way, because you have ten more years of life experience and personal growth to pull from to try an alternative path. It helps to know that we all go in circles, even when we think we're moving along a linear path. But now when your issues resurface, you truly have new skills—your mindfulness skills—to be able to go deeper.

Daily self-compassion is one of the most important aspects of this work. Sexuality is already so fraught with confusion and stigma, and female sexuality is shrouded in shame and disconnection. All meaningful personal growth challenges you to go to places you fear, and sexual personal growth takes this challenge to new depths. As I wrote in the Introduction, you must be willing to move toward your discomfort and pain, instead of away. Choosing this path certainly warrants more compassion for yourself. You are stronger than you think you are, and self-compassion is vital for your continuing strength and resiliency.

WHAT'S POSSIBLE

This book has covered so many of the negative aspects of our societal learnings about our bodies and sex. But once you realize that this doesn't have to be your truth, and that you can create a version of sexuality that fits your values and desires, you have opened endless doors of possibility. What is possible now? Here are some of the new experiences you may have after reading this book and committing to your action plan:

- ▸ Greater self-worth and knowing your value as a human
- ▸ Knowing that you are not alone with your sexual concerns
- ▸ Understanding that you are not broken
- ▸ Feeling proud of yourself for your open-mindedness to sexual exploration
- ▸ Having more awareness and joy in everyday moments
- ▸ Training your brain to work for you instead of against you
- ▸ Awareness of your patterns and an ability to kindly laugh at yourself when they surface
- ▸ Improved relationship communication and articulation of your needs
- ▸ Feeling proud that you are making healthy choices where once you were only reactive
- ▸ Experiencing the depth and beauty of vulnerability with another person
- ▸ Deeper appreciation for your partner and all they bring to your life
- ▸ Taking ownership of your desire
- ▸ Greater awareness and communication around your sexual fears
- ▸ Openness to learning new things about your body and how to experience pleasure
- ▸ More pleasure in sexual interactions
- ▸ Developing a creativity and playfulness around sexual interactions

- ▸ Embracing your body as your friend instead of your enemy
- ▸ Creating a version of feeling sexy that empowers you
- ▸ Taking more time for self-nurturing
- ▸ An ability to impact the sexuality of future generations of women in a positive way
- ▸ Viewing other women as sources of strength and connection, instead of competition
- ▸ Feeling inspired by your ability to make positive change in your own life
- ▸ Feeling a new vitality and passion for your life

Thank you for spending this time with me. I want to acknowledge you for your commitment to your sexual empowerment and your courage to create a new and authentic version of your sexual expression. And, as always, be kind to yourself.

ACKNOWLEDGMENTS

This—my first published book—is my baby. I want to thank all my friends and family who have continually treated me and my baby with kindness and encouragement.

I am so grateful that I've had the opportunity to work with Hannah Bennett as my editor at Cleis Press. You challenged me personally and professionally, and, although it made my brain hurt, I can't thank you enough for your gracious style and for making this book what I hoped it could be. Also, a generous thank you to the whole team at Cleis for your creativity and insights.

To my sex-field mentors, Patti Britton and the late Robert Dunlap and Gina Ogden: Thank you for your wisdom, support, and continued guidance on my path in this field. Sending big hugs and kisses!

I've had two interns over the years who assisted in this book. Thank you Roxana Torres Toreno and Ashley Labagnara for finding research articles and being my go-to people for random work requests. I also want to thank the thirty-five women who shared their stories about sex and gender roles with me back in 2007, and whose voices add candor and richness to chapter 6. And I am humbled by my clients whose struggles and successes inspired the examples I shared throughout this book.

Several friends stepped up to help by giving feedback on various chapters. Thank you Becca Karpinski, Sara Schairer, and Mary Williams for generously offering your time and your eyes of expertise. And thank you Anne Marie Welsh for seeing the potential in my book, for editing chapters and the proposal, and for guiding me through the somewhat painful process of learning how to write personal vignettes.

To my (mostly San Diego) friends, some who have heard about this book project for six plus years, you rock! Thank you to Karpo for your friendship and for our initial coaching sessions that kicked off this book. And deep gratitude to these friends for your support, laughter, meals, massages, brainstorming, and adventure: Elizabeth, Barb, Lyle, Rob, Sara, Heather, Sayaka, Chris, Sam, Liv, and Josh.

A big thank you to my big sister, Christine Gunsaullus, who edited a few of these chapters over the past few years and who has been my informal editor for many articles and blogs. I can't tell you how much it means to me to know that I can send a piece of writing to you and expect your insightful response within a mere few hours. You are an invaluable resource in my career and in my life. I feel lucky.

Finally, the immense appreciation I feel for my parents, Carol and Mike Gunsaullus, is beyond words. You have provided unconditional love and support through all my years of choosing not only a non-traditional path in life, but a non-traditional (and controversial) career as well. Your expression of pride in me makes me cry every time. Thank you—I wouldn't have this baby without you!